What's Next?

What's Next?

The Smart Nurse's Guide to Your Dream Job

How to Create a Personal Career Roadmap

Kati Kleber, BSN, RN, CCRN

American Nurses Association

Silver Spring, Maryland • 2016

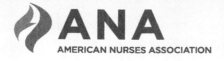

The America Nurses Association (ANA) is the premier organization representing the interests of the nation's 3.6 million registered nurses. ANA advances the nursing profession by fostering high standards of nursing practice, promoting a safe and ethical work environment, bolstering the health and wellness of nurses, and advocating on health care issues that affect nurses and the public. ANA is at the forefront of improving the quality of health care for all.

American Nurses Association
8515 Georgia Avenue, Suite 400
Silver Spring, MD 20910-3492
1-800-274-4ANA
http://www.Nursingworld.org

Library of Congress Cataloging-in-Publication data available on request.

978-1-55810-663-5 print   SAN: 851-3481   11/2016
978-1-55810-664-2 ePDF
978-1-55810-665-9 ePUB
978-1-55810-666-6 Kindle

First printing: November 2016

Contents

Author's Introduction: Finding Your Way to Your Dream Job and Career Path

Shining a Light on Nursing Professional Development

If you haven't realized it yet, the field of nursing is bigger than the endotracheal tubes used to sedate elephants for surgery: intimidating, very long, and leading into unlit spaces. When you see it, you don't even know where to start. The profession of nursing can be just like that. It offers so many different opportunities in different areas that it can be pretty daunting to attempt to make sense of it all. Following what your coworkers say or have done seems to be the only guide through this seemingly dark and unknown space. Maybe one coworker is nationally certified, another is a member of shared governance, and another is in graduate school. You are not sure what that all means, but they seem to enjoy what they are doing. However, they don't talk about it a whole lot and you don't want to seem clueless by asking basic questions.

Wanting answers to the basic questions about nursing professional development definitely does not classify anyone as clueless. There are many nurses who have been in the field for many years who still are not quite sure of all of the options, let alone how to maximize them. My hope is that this book will enable you to flip on the light switch to nursing professional development and turn those dark and unknown spaces into a brightly lit expanse in which you can pick and choose what you want to do and how you want to do it to find your way forward both professionally and personally.

While I was going to nursing school and for about a year after, I had no idea what else was out there within our profession beyond the bedside. I felt like I had to become very comfortable within my role as a bedside nurse before I could look further. Nursing school and being a new graduate is overwhelming enough. You are trying to absorb as much pertinent information as possible, as quickly as possible, to be able to safely care for patients. Professional development at this stage is not the priority because, even if you did have time, your brain is so overloaded with information that it is a challenge to remember to even do your own laundry, let alone really dive into perfecting your craft and learning more about your professional opportunities.

Where I'm Coming From: Why I Wrote This Book
I wrote this book because it took a lot of time for me to put the pieces of professional development together. It took me a while to fully understand all of the options and then figure out which was best for me at which points in my life. I asked a lot of questions, volunteered for various committees, took many classes, attended conferences, and paid attention when nurses did things well (like being a charge nurse, running a code, precepting a new graduate nurse, and so forth) and took note.

So why should you listen to me? Why should you care what I have to say? I know that to be trusted by nurses, one must prove oneself. It's like that brand new nurse to your unit who says they have experience within your specialty of nursing. While they say they know what they are talking about, you really have to see for yourself if they know what they are doing before you trust them fully with the patients who are so near and dear to you.

I get it and am a part of that mentality as well. I won't trust just anyone with my patients, nor will I take just anyone's advice on how to succeed in my career. So when the nurse that is new to our unit assures me she or he knows how to change a central line dressing, you better believe I watch them to make sure they know how to do it correctly. I don't know them from Adam, and I need to ensure that they know what they are doing.

My answer to that concern is this: I am a practicing bedside nurse. I am not far-removed from what it means to work at the bedside and also work on furthering my professional career. I understand the workload and stress you may be under, to a certain degree—I cannot claim that I know the ins and outs of all specialties in all areas. Everyone has their own kind of challenges, but I do know the general nurse struggle. I know what it feels like to hear three call lights going off in the background while you're trying to push dextrose as fast as possible into your hypoglycemic patient's IV with your hand shaking, see your other patient's blood pressure spike on the monitor, hear the phone ringing with two phone calls and no secretary, and know there's another patient's family member angrily waiting in the hallway to ask you why you haven't brought in their loved one's pain medication that you can't administer for 45 minutes anyway. I know what it feels like to come home from a day like that, because, while that was just the first 9 minutes of the shift, we all know it continues for the entirety of the 12 hours. It can feel like a punch in the gut to have days like that and be expected to care about professional development.

I get it. Because I understand that stress level, I get how precious your time is. This is a collection of the down and dirty basics of learning how to perfect your craft as a nurse. One could (and many have) write an entire nursing textbook about each chapter of this book. This is a starting-off point. This is the map of the whole country of nursing, and those books that go into more detail about the various aspects are the separate, more comprehensive maps of each important city. I have a list of recommended reading and other resources in the back of this book if you would like to dig deeper into the various topics.

I would also like to give you some more specifics about my career to strengthen my theoretical nurse soapbox. (If it's a nurse soapbox, it's probably an antimicrobial hand sanitizer box.) I obtained my BSN in May 2010 at Iowa Wesleyan University and have worked at the bedside since. I worked in a cardiovascular stepdown unit for the first two years and in neurosciences intensive care unit since. I have precepted new nurses for both critical care and stepdown units and taken multiple preceptor training courses at different facilities. I was precepted twice (once right out of school and again when I transitioned into critical care) by two very awesome, yet very different, well-rounded, and experienced preceptors. I completed a new-graduate residency at a Magnet®-designated facility. When I moved across the country, I began working at another Magnet hospital. I've been a member of shared governance at the unit, facility, and market levels of the corporation my hospital is a part of. Because of my shared governance experience, I have seen what it takes to build precepting programs, obtain a Magnet designation, initiate research studies, implement the latest evidence-based practice, and influence change from the perspective of a nurse administrator and also the end user: the bedside nurse.

I obtained my critical care certification from the American Association of Critical Care Nurses in 2015. I've authored two books in addition to this one, one for nursing students and new grads and another for patients. I've been writing a blog for prospective nurses, nursing students, new grads, and seasoned nurses since 2013, curating the information I've learned over the years so others don't have to make the same mistakes I've made or take as long to figure things out.

Where You Might Be Going: Why This Book Could Be For You

Before going into the details however, I want you to know that as a nurse at this particular point in your career (that period when you feel very comfortable in your role as a nurse; typically after two years), you are powerful. I first discuss why this moment is extremely pivotal in your career. I then go into details about some of the more practical advice for successfully evolving into a formal or informal nurse on your unit, from learning how to be an effective charge nurse to how to precept and mentor new nurses. I then go into the details that are behind providing better or more effective bedside care. I outline what going to graduate school in the field of nursing really looks like, and how professional organizations, certifications, and conferences can help you take your career beyond the bedside. I also discuss what shared governance and the Magnet designation actually mean from a bedside, administrative, and patient perspective.

While my personal experience is limited to stepdown and critical care nursing, this information is applicable to most areas of our field: from the labor and delivery nurse aspiring to become a midwife, to the US Army vet working in the ER, to the school nurse working at an elementary school in rural Iowa. Maybe you are not in the position to ever be a charge nurse or team leader of a unit of 15+ nurses, but you most likely will be in a position to lead others, and the information in Chapter 2 can be applicable to those situations as well.

Nurses, from all areas of the field, are powerful people, but we have to understand the resources that are available and their importance to really harness that power to maximize both our experience and our patients'. I hope this book helps you switch on your own source of light and find your way to the next steps of your nursing career. May it make those dark and unknown areas of our field not only visible but something you want to be a part of. In my case, I think the light bulbs that first showed me my way through nursing professional development were those energy-conserving light bulbs; it took a long time for them to light up and for everything to become visible and clear to me. While I used to believe that being a competent bedside nurse was the end-all goal, I have since learned that it is only the beginning.

Author's Disclaimer

The information and examples in this book are for informational purposes only. Always follow your facility's policies and procedures when providing direct patient care, and direct any questions, comments, or concerns through the chain of command established at your facility. Please refer to your respective state board of nursing for information and rules regarding the varying levels of nursing school and for questions related to licensure. The views and experiences in this book do not reflect any past or current employers, coworkers, patients, or their loved ones. All patient examples mentioned in this book are fictional or hypothetical.

1

Presenting Two Career Paths: The Power of the Advanced Beginner

You feel like you have finally made it. You no longer feel anxiety before you walk onto the unit. You are pretty confident that you can handle most situations that come your way, and for those that you don't know how to handle, you know who to call. You've made friends on the unit. The doctors, nurse practitioners, and physician assistants know you. At least one or two more nurses have started after you, so you feel like you can be a resource to them. People come to you with questions and you know the answers. You feel like you belong.

This is the feeling you have been waiting for since you walked into your first nursing course. This is it.

While you may not realize it, this is a pivotal time in your nursing career. As an advanced beginner, you have a lot of influence over the culture of a nursing unit, and this time of your career is essential. You're out from under the wings of a preceptor. You still talk to your mentor regularly, but your relationship has evolved into more of a professional friendship than a mentor–mentee relationship. You are starting to feel like equals. You're developing your own nursing identity outside the influence of your coworkers, who are deeply rooted in both their own routines and who they are as nurses.

Two Nursing Career Paths
The Complacent Path
As I previously stated, this period of time is crucial. There are two paths in front of you. I like to call one of these two paths the *Complacent Path*. In this path, you'll mold yourself to the other complacent nurses on the unit. Going to work becomes only that: work. You will clock in, do the minimum of what is expected, and then go home. You'll complete your education on time, but you won't volunteer for any committees. You will still care for your patients, but you will soon find yourself on autopilot. You always want call time, you always want to go home early, and if you have to float to another unit, you'll complain for the entire shift and the next three thereafter.

Change, which is inevitable in this profession, will ruffle your feathers. You'll feel like Donald Duck after a hurricane. It will cause you to complain and commiserate with the other complacent nurses on your unit. Even though you won't realize it, it will profoundly affect the culture. This will eventually mold you into the nurse who is never happy. Because you're no longer being challenged, because it has become only about the tasks in front of you and not the bigger picture of nursing, you will get bored. You've learned what you need to know to do your job, so you are now complacent. While you will learn new things every so often, it won't be the same as being consistently challenged and invigorated.

Things that go wrong will inevitably be the fault of the patient, the family, or your employer. When someone or something does not go right, the routine is to complain until it blows over. The ability to understand the other side of things, the grace, and the kindness you once had will dwindle. You may still feel these things, but you will have created this image within the culture of your unit. A tough, powerful image. You won't be able to break that within your group of complacency nurses. That would be heresy.

It's hard to break from this path. It's hard to find joy in this career once you've been down it for so many years, especially if you've been on the same unit and have a deeply rooted reputation.

The Challenge Me Path

But, there is another option, another path. I call this the *Challenge Me Path*. At this pivotal time in your career when you finally feel like you have your feet under you, you won't be satisfied. You will want to know and learn more. Now that you can manage a major task list without thinking about it, now that you can see what working at the bedside really looks like and means, you will want to understand more. You will want to be aware of what's behind the scenes, why we do what we do, and have a say in it.

Now that you don't come home every night completely emotionally exhausted shift after shift, you will be able to think about what else you want from your career. You'll look at those positive nurses who have formal and informal leadership roles and want what they have. You will start to formulate your next goal.

You may volunteer to do some chart audits, ask to be trained to be a preceptor, or cross-train in similar units or for specific procedures or patients that are more complex. You may ask to be a part of shared governance (I'll talk more about this later) or offer to help someone with a research project. You will begin to understand the bigger picture of being a nurse. You will walk into work each day with more understanding and a softer heart. When change occurs, you will look at it objectively instead of immediately picking apart the flaws.

This will spill over into your patient care. You will be able to empathize with patients on a different level. You will never get bored or tired of this because it will continually challenge you, not only making you a better nurse but a better person.

I want you to think about the nurses on your unit. Think about how long they've been on your particular unit, when they may have hit this cross-roads, and which path they chose to take. What do you think about them as a nurse now? Are they technically proficient, safe, or even advanced? Are they understanding of each patient and their specific needs? Are they quick to judge or quick to listen? When change occurs, how do they respond? Do they take accountability for their actions, or do they quickly divert blame?

These things I've pointed out are not always apparent. Some nurses make a wonderful first impression, but farther down the line, you realize how unhappy, complacent, or even angry they are inside. This is something that can even be difficult to notice about yourself, if you're not honest. My challenge to you, when you are at this critical moment in your career, is to examine what you want out of nursing. Is this now, and has it always been, just a job and way to earn money? Or is there something deeper to this career that you appreciate and enjoy?

With this active decision, not only do you to have the power to profoundly influence your personal future, but also the culture of the unit. I have seen complacent nurses utterly destroy a unit, to the point where patients and families can feel their lack of caring. Conversely, I have seen engaged and caring nurses elevate a nursing unit so far that they set the standard very high for their new hires and patient satisfaction scores were off the charts.

Sometimes, all a unit needs are some nurses who are not afraid to say no to complacency. Nurses who will boldly and unapologetically put their own personal and professional career development ahead of being best buds with the strongest personalities on the unit. You can make this transition at any time during your career, but I argue that it is easiest to do so as an advanced beginner.

If you are taking the time to get deeper into your career, others will notice. Others will see how you respond to situations. If there is an opportunity to complain about something and you do not take it, people notice. If, when others want to talk negatively about a coworker, you choose not to respond, bring to light positive things about that employee, or just exit the conversation, again, people will notice.

You may not be able to tell when people take note, but they will. The people this makes a deep impression on are the brand new employees, experienced or not. They learn that they do not have to commiserate to fit in. Creating a culture in which people do not bond or develop friendships on the basis of complaining or gossiping is tougher than one might think, but it is possible.

The priority of the informal leaders on the unit cannot be complaining and gossiping. This is the cancer of the unit. New employees long to fit in and bond with new coworkers, and if the only way to do this is to make fun of others or complain about the new enteral feeding policy, pretty soon that will be the foundation of the unit. To fit in, to belong, to be a part of the team, they will have to be negative. Soon, people who are not negative or gossipy will become that way as a survival tactic.

What results from this survival tactic are people who commiserate so that they will have some friends at work. They'll have people to rely on when suddenly they are overwhelmed or they need help with their patients, so they don't get stranded when they need it most. It may not be a way they would act normally, but it's what they have to do to not be the outcast, left to fend for themselves.

But you, oh advanced beginner, you have the power to change this or prevent this from happening. You are an informal leader, my friend. Whether you realize it or not, you are someone others will go to for questions, someone others look up to. New nurses, new nursing aides, or even nurses with more experience but have just started working in your unit will look to you for guidance. They will ask you questions, but they will observe your behavior as well. And how you carry yourself, how you respond to patients, how you react to change, how you handle criticism and correction often times stays in their memory much longer and has a much bigger impact than the personal conversations you have with them.

Yes, people are watching.

In this book, I will discuss how you can optimize the *Challenge Me Path* of nursing. My hope and prayer is that this will enable you not only to be a better nurse, but also to discover a new level of personal and professional job satisfaction. You are worth that, your patients are worth that, and you have the power to profoundly impact this profession.

2

Learning How To Be a Charge Nurse: Some "Challenge Me" Scenarios

Many times, once you have shown competency in your nursing care, management will look to train you to be in charge of the unit. I have been in charge and also worked under many different charge nurses.

Please note, many hospitals handle this role differently and call the role something other than charge nurse. Some facilities call this role a team lead, the lead nurse, etc. Some facilities allow the nurse in charge not to have a patient assignment; some give this nurse a smaller assignment; some assign this nurse the same number of patients but with a lower acuity; and some give this nurse a full patient load.

For the basic purpose of understanding, I will utilize the term "charge nurse" and assume this person has a patient load with fewer patients than the rest of the nurses. Again, I realize this is not always the case, but to explain some helpful hints and tricks, I will go under this assumption.

Responsibilities of the charge nurse also differ from facility to facility. These can include, but are not limited to: creating the patient assignment for the next shift, facilitating patient flow in and out of the unit, dealing with any medical emergencies, touching base with management, addressing customer service–related issues, facilitating communication with members of the medical team when there are concerns or issues, assigning patients to nurses as they come to the unit, and various tasks from management (for example, ensuring people have completed various educational requirements or specific charting).

The last, yet probably most important aspect of this role is being the leader of the unit for the next 12 hours. You are the go-to person when the nurses, physicians, patients, families, management, and others have a question or concern. You are looked at as a resource. This does not mean you know all of the answers, but you know many of them, and for the questions you don't know the answers, you know who to call.

Typically, when you are chosen for this role, it is because you have gotten to a point where you can confidently handle your patient assignment with ease. You clock in, get your assignment, do a good job, and clock out on time. You do not get overwhelmed or frazzled when things start to go downhill. You are familiar with the processes of the hospital, how patients are admitted, discharged, and transferred. You are aware of most of the hospital's resources. You are also extremely familiar with your patient population.

Your colleagues feel comfortable and confident in your knowledge base. They consider you a source of information regarding nursing care. They bounce things off you before calling the physician. They trust your judgment.

I have had the pleasure of working under many different charge nurses throughout my career. Some had great leadership and time management skills, and some did not. I am going to walk through a 12-hour shift and present you with how a good charge nurse (Nurse Awesome, who will be male) would handle this situation versus how a bad charge nurse (Nurse Blah, who will also be male) would handle it. First, I will outline some important guidelines and then illustrate their importance with a scenario.

Let's go!

Scene

We are in a 25-bed intermediate unit, and this is day shift. Shift change is from 0700–0730 (and 1900–1930). The unit currently has 20 patients. Three nurses have 4 patients, two have 3 patients, and the charge nurse has 2 patients. There are two CNAs and one medical unit secretary. One nurse is floating to a medical–surgical (med–surg) unit.

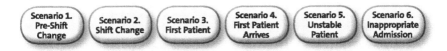

Scenario 1. Pre-Shift Change

Time: 0645

Arrive early. Get your mind around the day. Understand which patients are not doing well, who will be discharged or transferred, which nurses will get the first few admissions, and so on. If possible, know what days you'll be in charge so you can mentally prepare yourself before coming in. If someone has to float, you should be aware early to let them know as soon as they arrive. Some people really hate floating to another unit, but it's part of the job. Go by whatever process your unit has developed, do not play favorites, and communicate professionally, appropriately, and promptly.

Nurse Awesome He walks on the unit, finishing up his coffee. He's ready to go. He greets the previous shift and touches base with the previous charge nurse about how the night went and what today will look like. He checks the assignment and sees who his patients are. He takes notes on what the previous charge nurse told him and starts looking up information about his patients. He decides, based on number of patients and acuity, who will get the first few admissions. He also makes sure he knows which patients are not doing so hot and who to keep an eye on.

Lisa shows up, and he tells her that she's floating. She's not happy, but it's her turn and he makes sure she's aware of that. She openly asks the new nurses in the nurse's station to float for her, but Nurse Awesome interjects and tells her that it's her turn and they've already gotten their assignments. They're secretly extremely relieved and thankful he said something, since she's a strong personality and they're new and don't want to ruffle any feathers.

Nurse Blah He's not here yet. Lisa waits to get her assignment for ten minutes but doesn't know she is floating because the night shift charge nurse is already in report. She's late to get report on the medical–surgical unit and walks off frustrated. She would have tried to pawn off her float day on some new nurse, but everyone is already in report so it's too late.

Scenario 2. Shift Change
Time: 0700

Communicate with the team. Preemptively inform them who will be the first person to get an admission. The worst way to handle this is by asking, "Who wants to take the next patient?" Newsflash: No one does. Handle this fairly and in a matter-of-fact way. Some nurses will act like you're just trying to make their day worse by giving them a patient, but this is just part of the job.

Nurse Awesome Now that he has his head around what today will look like, he is ready to greet the masses. He gathers the oncoming nurses and CNAs for a quick good morning and pep talk.

"Good morning, everyone. We are at 20 patients. The ICUs may have 4–5 transfers out early because they have a few surgeries on today. Lisa floated to med–surg today, so if we get slammed, I'll try to get her back. Kayla, you will take the first transfer or admit, and Travis, you'll take the second. If you get transfer orders early, I would hop on them because we all know the ICU will be calling soon to clear out. Tomorrow is the last day for the glucose meter update, so make sure you get that done if you haven't already. Also, there are a lot of contact-isolation patients today. So, CNAs, if you could keep the gowns and gloves outside of the room stocked, I'd really appreciate it. Ok, let me know if you need anything. I have beds 88 and 89."

He then goes to get report from the night shift nurses on his two patients.

Nurse Blah He clocks in at 0659 and doesn't say a word until 0705. (You know, he's got to finish his coffee.) He didn't realize he was in charge today. He's annoyed that he's got to do that as well as take care of patients. He tries to find the night shift charge nurse, but she's already giving report to the oncoming nurse because shift change has already started. He sits and waits for her.

It's 0715, and he still doesn't know anything. The night shift charge nurse surfaces, and she gives him the rundown of the night before. He's excited Travis and Kayla are working today because they're good friends. Plus they only have three patients each, so they'll be able to hang out a bit since they don't have a full load.

He doesn't do morning huddles or announcements. It's not his thing. Everyone is scattered, getting report. He goes and gets report on his two patients, and it's about 0745 before he even starts his day.

Scenario 3. The First Patient
Time: 0852

Do not play favorites. Even if you think you're being nice to your buds, everyone else hates it. This does not foster a team who wants to work together and help each other out. This creates cliques, frustration, and resentment. Gossip results. It is not a good idea, ever, to play favorites or give your buds an easier day. Treat everyone fairly, regardless of how nice they are to you or how close your friendship may be outside of work. You do not want to enable one another.

Help people out consistently throughout the day. If you're caught up, check on everyone. See what you can do to help them. If you know a coworker is getting a patient and you're doing okay, make sure they are ready. Keeping people on time or ahead of schedule means they're not as overwhelmed. They'll be willing to help others if they know you've got their back. Help get rooms ready, start IVs, answer call lights and IV pumps, etc.

Nurse Awesome The phone rings, and the unit is getting a patient from the ICU. Nurse Awesome assigns the bed and goes to let Kayla know. She was trying to hustle a little this morning because she knew she would get the first patient. He asks her if she needs help getting anything done before she gets report, since it's med pass time. She says she is almost done with her meds, but she just hasn't charted anything. Nurse Awesome has already seen, charted, and given his patients their meds, so he finishes her meds so she can get caught up before report. Kayla goes to the nurse's station to chart until the ICU calls report.

On his way back to the nurse's station, Nurse Awesome peeks into the room that the patient will be going to, to make sure it's set up. He double checks that the bed is zeroed and gets a few things out he knows Kayla will need. He informs Marsha, the CNA for Kayla, that she's going to be getting a patient in the near future and that the room is ready to go.

After Kayla gets report, he asks her to tell him a little about the patient so he's aware of what to expect. They have a tracheostomy and are on contact isolation for MRSA. He goes to get the contact-isolation signs and cart and double checks that suction is set up.

Nurse Blah The phone rings, and the unit is getting a patient from the ICU. He doesn't know who is up for the next patient, so he goes to check the board. It's Travis or Kayla, his buds. He likes to be able to help them out when he's working to make sure they have a good day. He sees what other nurses have for an assignment to see if he can give this patient to someone else.

He sees Marissa at the nurse's station. She was here yesterday, knows her patients pretty well, and is a pretty efficient nurse. He thinks she might agree to take this patient, so he might as well try. He asks her and she reluctantly says yes, even though she has a full load already. A few minutes later she realizes that both Kayla and Travis are open for admissions. This makes her pretty frustrated, and she musters up the courage to go ask him why Travis or Kayla aren't getting these patients. "Umm, well they both have heavier patients than you, and you were already caught up," Nurse Blah says.

"You know I'm caught up because I was here yesterday, and nothing has changed with my patients. It is still a full load, and they both have room to admit," Marissa firmly says.

"Ok fine, I'll give it to one of them," Nurse Blah replies.

Tension is high. Marissa is upset; she goes and talks to another nurse about it. She thinks Kayla or Travis may have put him up to it. This is not a good way to start the day.

Nurse Blah goes to find Kayla to tell her she's getting the next patient. She kind of figured since she only had three patients to start out with. Because he wasted time trying to help out his friends, Kayla didn't have much warning before report was waiting on the phone for her. She's in the middle of passing meds, and she hasn't charted on her other patients. She's already behind, and she's getting another patient. Nurse Blah walks back to the nurse's station without offering to help her.

He doesn't check the room, and he doesn't touch base with the CNA, who is giving a bath to another patient. He sees Travis in the hallway and stops to chat for four to seven minutes.

Scenario 4. The First Patient Arrives
Time: 0917

Be proactive, not reactive. Prepare for incoming patients, anticipate their needs, and get things set up or ready for their arrival. It will make their transition much smoother and therefore make everyone's job easier.

Other ways to be proactive include knowing which patients will be the first to be triaged out when the unit is full and there are surgeries scheduled. It is much easier to be aware of this and communicate with physicians early to facilitate transfers or discharges than to frantically move patients later. Situations like that don't need to be emergencies, but they can turn into them quickly.

Additionally, if you know a family or patient is upset about something, randomly go check on them to see if they need anything. This can simmer a situation and prevent people from blowing up. Again, avoiding a crisis or emergent situation is always preferred!

Communicate with the team. The key to being proactive is communication. I cannot stress this enough. You can't be proactive if you're not talking to your team to see what kind of patient is on the way, who is overwhelmed, who is confused, or if someone is having problems getting what they need from the physician for their patient. You will find yourself putting out fires and doing more work than necessary. You will also find your staff members getting frustrated and falling behind. If they are overwhelmed all day because you did not communicate so they could not prepare, people will dread the days you are in charge.

Never blame your coworkers for lapses in customer service to save face. Maybe things could have been handled better, but transferring blame and not holding yourself accountable for things to patients and families is a poor way to handle yourself. If you made a mistake and owe a patient or loved one an apology, apologize. It is okay to say you're sorry.

Nurse Awesome He sees the patient rolling down the hallway, so he finds Kayla in one of her patient rooms and lets her know they've arrived. He also lets the CNA, Marsha, know as well, and meets the new patient in the room. While waiting for Kayla and Marsha to finish up what they are doing, Nurse Awesome helps settle the patient. He asks the medical unit secretary to direct the family to the waiting room.

They get the patient on the bed and comfortable and Kayla assesses her patient. Both the secretary and the CNA knew the patient was coming, so they are already transferred in the computer and the CNA is ready to hook the patient up to the monitor and label everything.

While Kayla is assessing the patient, Nurse Awesome gets the family and gives them a little information about the unit. After the new patient and family are settled, Nurse Awesome checks on his two patients.

Nurse Blah He sees the patient rolling down the hallway. He waits until he sees them enter the room before he gets up. He goes to tell Kayla and Marsha their patient has arrived. Marsha had no idea, and she's in the middle of a bed bath with a high fall risk patient whom she cannot leave alone. She would not have started this bath if she had known she was getting a patient. She's frustrated that Nurse Blah didn't give her a heads up at all. Kayla is frantically finishing her last meds in another room. It takes her 4 minutes to get there.

Nurse Blah goes back to the nurse's station. He figures that between the ICU nurse who brought the patient, Marsha, and Kayla, they won't need any help. He doesn't ask or check.

The ICU nurse waits patiently with the patient and their family in the room. Finally Kayla arrives. Marsha is tied up, so Kayla goes up to the nurse's station to get Nurse Blah who slowly walks to the room. Kayla asks the family to go to the waiting room. It takes her about 5 minutes to show them where it is and get back. They finally get the patient settled. The ICU nurse is frustrated because he has an unstable patient on the way from the OR, and it's taken him 20 minutes to transfer a patient when it should have taken 6 minutes.

Kayla is trying to assess the patient, hook him up to the monitor, and label everything alone. Nurse Blah is already sitting back down in the nurse's station, checking Facebook on his phone, and Marsha is still giving the bath.

Kayla finally finishes and goes to get the family. They're frustrated it took so long to get him settled, but she didn't have any help and honestly didn't want to ask Nurse Blah for help anyway. He would have taken forever to get to the room, completed tasks slowly, and been more of a bother than help because he'd want to chat.

Scenario 5. The Unstable Patient
Time: 1012

Do what the unit needs most, not what you enjoy most. Being in charge doesn't mean you get to call all the shots and everyone does what you say. It doesn't mean you get to put your feet up at the nurse's station just to be "available" if needed, while everyone else runs around like crazy. That is not your job. Your job is to ensure the patients get the best care possible and ensure the unit runs smoothly. If a patient is deteriorating, their primary nurse needs to be available to address it and take control. You are there to assist in whatever they need, not to run the show. Also, if you are all caught up, it's not time to take a break. Your responsibility is to ensure the unit as a whole is functioning and running well, and you can't do that if you take a coffee break every 20 minutes and chat for 45 minutes with every doctor who rounds. Check on your nurses and CNAs and see what tasks you can do to get everyone in a good place.

Nurse Awesome At the beginning of the shift, the night shift charge nurse let him know that the patient in room 67 didn't have a great night.

He's getting two units of blood right now. He's got a GI bleed, but the night nurse was worried he was developing sepsis. The night nurse told the doc about the concerns, but they didn't feel an ICU transfer was necessary. Since the blood has been administered, he's been doing a bit better. Since he was already aware of this situation, Nurse Awesome has been making sure the nurse caring for this patient has been doing okay. He checks on the patient and asks how he can help the nurse. She's a little concerned as well.

The patient's stool had been dark red and solid. They think his bleed has been resolving, as his H/H has steadily been increasing. However, the CNA just put him on the bedpan and he had a large, liquid, bright red bowel movement that looked like straight blood. She immediately called for help. The nurse and Nurse Awesome get there immediately. His blood pressure is 78/40, pulse 129; he's pale, stuporous, and diaphoretic. Nurse Awesome calls the rapid response nurse (resource nurse, code nurse, or whatever your facility may call it) for an extra set of hands; he then runs to get fluid and supplies for lab draws. While the patient's nurse is assessing him, giving him fluid, and putting him in reverse Trendelenburg, Nurse Awesome has the secretary STAT page the MD. The rapid response nurse arrives and, along with the primary nurse, gives him some fluid, puts in another IV, draws some labs, and arranges a transfer to the ICU. Nurse Awesome works to facilitate the transfer while the nurse is with the patient and the MD, who just arrived.

The patient is transferred immediately with the code nurse and the patient's nurse. Nurse Awesome calls the family at home to let them know what happened. When he's done with that, he goes to check on the nurse's other patients and sees if they need any meds since she'll be gone about 20 minutes probably.

This started going downhill at 1012, and the patient got to ICU at 1052.

Nurse Blah The above scenario starts to unfold. However, Nurse Blah has no idea that one patient didn't look so great. When he hears the CNA yell for help, he runs into the room. He doesn't know what's going on at all with this patient, but he correctly assumes a GI bleed. He gets into "go-time mode" and starts to assess the patient, check vitals, and so on. The patient's nurse arrives shortly thereafter, and he starts asking her tons of questions. She's trying to address the situation and answer his basic questions simultaneously. Minutes later, after he understands the situation, he tells her to call the doctor.

She leaves the room to do so. He's taken over for all the tasks and starts telling people what to do. While they are the correct things, people aren't working together to get things accomplished or assessed, so it takes longer and is much more inefficient.

While on the phone, the doctor tells the nurse that the patient should probably go to the ICU. He gives her orders for labs, fluid, etc.

The nurse comes back to the room to tell Nurse Blah. He tells her to call rapid response to take care of the transfer and to go get him stuff to draw labs and give fluid immediately. She complies, and he stays at the bedside, taking care of her patient. He loves taking care of unstable patients and would rather do that than run around anyway.

The MD and rapid response nurse get to the bedside and start asking questions that he's not equipped to answer. The patient's nurse is, but she's running around gathering supplies and making calls. They have to wait for her to arrive to get a better picture of what's going on. The rapid response nurse starts giving him fluid once the patient's nurse arrives with it while Nurse Blah pulls blood for labs and starts an IV. The patient's nurse talks to the MD, then Nurse Blah tells her to call the supervisor to facilitate the transfer to the ICU. She does so, again, taking her away from the bedside and leaving him there.

The transfer is facilitated, and she is packing the patient up to take him to the ICU with the rapid response nurse. Nurse Blah insists on coming, even though it would be more beneficial for him to stay back and not take two nurses off the floor. He loves the ICU and goes any chance he gets. They arrive in the ICU, and the patient's nurse gives the ICU nurse report while Nurse Blah chats it up with a few ICU nurses.

This started at 1012, and the patient arrived in the ICU at 1117.

The patient's nurse hurries to get back because she's already behind with her other patients since this all went down. Nurse Blah hangs out in the ICU for about 20 minutes.

The nurse is frantically charting what just happened, checking her patients, and getting their meds. Nurse Blah slowly walks back to the nurse's desk. He recently checked on his patients, so he doesn't feel the need to go see them again right now. The family of the patient that just got transferred runs up to the nurse's station, "Where's my dad? He was just in that room and now it's empty! Did something happen?!"

"Oh," says Nurse Blah. "The nurse should have called you immediately. We had to transfer him to the ICU. I'll go get her so she can give you an update." He walks to go get her, leaving the family a nervous, crying wreck.

When the nurse arrives to talk to them, she immediately apologizes for not calling, and they are furious. "It's her problem, not mine," Nurse Blah thinks, as he sends Travis a text to see if he wants to go to lunch. The nurse is frustrated by the lack of support and leadership, and that she is being thrown under the bus and completely overwhelmed while he's just hanging out.

Scenario 6. The Inappropriate Admission
Time: 1501

Learn about each new patient the unit will be receiving. Sometimes a patient is set to come to your unit that should not be. It takes a nurse who is familiar with the unit, its processes, and its patient population to ensure that only the correct and appropriate patients are coming to the unit. Every time you get report, find out a little bit about the patient.

Nurse Awesome Another patient is coming up, this time from the Emergency Department. Latisha knew she was up for the next admission so she was ready for report. After the nurse finished getting report, Nurse Awesome touches base with Latisha about the patient. This nurse just got off orientation and is doing great, but she has not been here very long, so she's not extremely familiar with all of the processes of the hospital.

"They're completely stable but on a Cardizem drip for atrial fibrillation," she tells Nurse Awesome.

"Interesting," he says. "That sounds like a patient that doesn't necessarily need to come to us. The cardiac unit sounds like a more appropriate place for this patient. I'm going to double check the chart and call the house supervisor to let them know. They just changed it so that the cardiac floor can take Cardizem drips, and I wonder if that ED doc just didn't know of the change."

He calls the house supervisor, who speaks with the physician in the emergency department. He was not aware of the change, and agrees that the patient would be more appropriate for the other unit. They decide to send this patient to the cardiac floor instead.

Report was given at 1501, the transfer was changed at 1511.

Nurse Blah Another patient is coming. He tells Latisha, who is giving a patient medications, that she's getting a patient and that report is on the phone. She is frustrated that she had no idea she was next and now has to drop everything to get report. She frantically finishes giving this patient medications while the Emergency Department nurse is stuck on hold for 10 minutes, getting frustrated.

Latisha gets report. Nurse Blah gets himself more coffee.

The patient arrives on the unit, and the nurse and her CNA get the patient settled. Nurse Blah doesn't really notice they've arrived. After she finishes settling him, she goes up to the nurse's desk to ask the secretary to get him into the system, since Nurse Blah didn't facilitate this. Jay, another nurse, asks her what's the deal with the new patient. She tells him that the patient is totally fine and just on a Cardizem drip and they should be an easy patient.

"That sounds like a patient for the cardiac floor, not our floor," Jay says.

"Oh, I had no idea. I'm still getting used to your patient population here," Latisha says.

"No big deal," he says. "They changed which floors can take which drips recently and the cardiac floor can take patients on Cardizem. Nurse Blah, didn't you know that?"

"Um. Yeah. I did, but I didn't know that's what was going on with this patient. Why didn't anyone tell me?" says Nurse Blah.

"I didn't know I needed to tell you, and you didn't ask me. I just assumed that was a normal patient for this unit," Latisha says.

"Okay, I'll call supervision," says Nurse Blah.

Sure enough, the patient should not have come to this unit. Supervision facilitates the transfer to the cardiac floor. The nurse informs the patient and their family, who are upset they are moving rooms since they were in the emergency department for six hours already.

The nurse gives report and transfers the patient to the correct room.

Report was given at 1511, and the patient finally arrives in the correct room at 1707. The cardiac floor was planning their assignment for the night shift already and has to change everything now to accommodate this additional patient.

Approaches to Being an In-Charge Nurse

You can see that there are different ways to approach being in charge. Being a good leader encompasses anticipation, preparation, and an ability to see how the entire unit functions rather than to simply view each nurse and her or his patients all in their own little silos.

An important part of all of this is being someone whom the staff feels comfortable going to with questions or concerns. They know you won't make them feel stupid for asking a remedial question or you won't go talk about them to your friends on the unit. It is important to be professional, appropriate, approachable, and encouraging. If your unit is intimidated by you, they are much less likely to come to you when they need something or when they're concerned. You'll find yourself dealing with a lot more emergencies because people didn't want to bring something to you unless they absolutely had to.

Additionally, it's important to handle staff issues appropriately and professionally. If you can see two staff members are mad at each other, see if you can get them to chat in a private area instead of complaining about each other to others. I know people typically don't want to get involved if they don't have to, but a strong leader will step in and privately mediate the situation. Also, if you notice someone isn't pulling their weight (others are answering all of their alarms, call lights, IV pumps, and so on while they chat with their buds), it is your job to say something. Pull them aside into a private area, and address it with them professionally. They may be frustrated with you, but the rest of the unit will rejoice and sing your praises. Nipping this in the bud is essential to maintaining an efficient and effective nursing unit with happy nurses.

Some assume that it is the manager's responsibility to address these concerns; however, that is unnecessary. Rarely is the manager there to observe this behavior first-hand and correct it in the moment. These situations are best addressed colleague-to-colleague, peer-to-peer as they occur. As professional nurses, we must hold each other accountable and therefore create a culture in which we can provide constructive criticism and have crucial conversations without taking things personally. This is an essential aspect of a healthy unit culture. Managers can step in if a mediator is necessary; however, this should be the exception and not the rule.

It's also important that you keep your opinions of the staff to yourself. Maybe the new girl is needy, and the guy that's been here for 10 years is lazy, and the CNA is rude, but that doesn't mean you need to talk about it. If it truly is an issue that is negatively impacting patients, they should be spoken to about the concern. When people hear you complain or talk negatively about others, they automatically think, "If they're saying this about someone else, I wonder what they say about me when I'm not around?" This promotes a very unhealthy culture. Model respectful behavior, and do not engage in unit gossip.

Being in charge can sound intimidating at first, but once you learn the ropes, you'll be a pro before you know it! There's something satisfying about being the go-to person on the unit. It can be quite the confidence builder and challenge you to be better. If you make it a point to be a proactive leader who communicates effectively and supports your team, you will soon be the charge nurse that people are happy to see when they walk on the unit. People will want to work hard for you. They will want to provide amazing patient care because you set the example. Even some of the toughest shifts will be manageable because of your leadership.

3

Becoming an Awesome Preceptor: Orienting the Newbies

I was very fortunate to have some amazing preceptors both when I started floor nursing and again when I transitioned into critical care. I've also had the privilege of precepting people in both areas. I pray I was a tiny fraction as awesome as my preceptors were to me. Many people assume that you have to be a nurse with extensive experience to train others. However, sometimes the best preceptors are those that have advanced past advanced beginners and are now competent in their clinical role. Nurses at this stage of development are keenly aware of policies, procedures, and regulations and went through orientation only a few years prior, rather than a few decades prior. They are able to relate well to the brand-new nurse.

What's a Preceptor?
Before we dive into how to be a successful preceptor, it's essential that to clearly understand the term. Many believe that a nurse preceptor is merely the person who trains a new nurse during the orientation phase. However, this position requires much more than just showing someone how to complete tasks. A nurse preceptor educates the new hire about all of the intricacies involved in becoming a safe care provider—a task that in itself is

an inch wide and a mile deep—and helps socialize them into the culture of the unit and facility. And serves as a role model. Yes; all that.

Nurse preceptors are responsible for ensuring the new hire understands policies and procedures, for holding them accountable when mistakes are made, and for providing education to fill in the gaps. They keep a close and continual eye on the educational needs throughout orientation to ensure the new hire has ample opportunity to experience as many scenarios and patient cases as possible.

Nurse preceptors also work closely with management to provide updates on the progression of orientation: if there are concerns about lack of progression, they can provide insights and help troubleshoot the situation. While often preceptors and preceptees become well acquainted, with friendships developing, the relationship should remain somewhat formal and structured to ensure that accountability remains consistent.

The process of successfully training a new nurse can be quite labor-intensive, but if you understand where they are in their development as a nurse as well as the general structure for the orientation process, it will make this very comprehensive and detailed task much more manageable.

I will first explain some important things to know about precepting in general and then go into the specifics of the different phases of nursing orientation.

Task-Focused Nurses

Something to keep in mind is that your newbies will be entirely task-focused. What I mean by task-focused is that they will be worrying about completing the list of tasks you give them rather than which to do first, the most efficient order in which to address them, and red flags. Things that may seem obvious to you might not be to them at this point. They'll be figuring out how to use the IV pumps, how to hook up the heart monitor, meeting the staff, discovering the location of every little thing, and so on. While it might be obvious to you to first delegate taking a patient to the bathroom so you can start a heparin drip, your orientee may gravitate toward helping the patient to the bathroom first because they're more comfortable with that, even though it's not the priority.

This is normal. As you are facing these various prioritization dilemmas, use these instances as teaching opportunities. "Tell me what you were thinking when you decided to do that first," is something I like to ask. You want them to think about why they're doing these specific things. You don't want them to just put their head down and complete as many tasks possible in the shortest amount of time. You want them to think about why they're choosing to do specific tasks first. This will enable them to troubleshoot better later on and develop their critical thinking skills.

Additionally, newer nurses typically are not that comfortable with delegation yet. It can be tough delegating to CNAs who have worked on this unit for 15 years when they just started last week. It's understandably challenging. The tendency is to do as much yourself without having to ask others. This mentality needs to be addressed as soon as it's noticed because it is incredibly inefficient. Here is how I would respond in the above situation:

"I can see you're going to take that patient to the bathroom first. Tell me why you're thinking of doing that task first." (Wait for response.) "Here is how I would attack this: I would delegate taking Mr. Smith to the bathroom to the CNA who is charting. Then that would allow me to start my heparin drip. If I couldn't remember exactly how to start that drip, I would look up the policy."

Again, this is how it should start. You will add the critical thinking piece later. You don't want them to feel like you're picking apart every little thing they're doing, but you want them to develop good and effective prioritization skills, which will make them extremely efficient and therefore productive.

Your Attitude as a Preceptor

One thing to be aware of is your attitude while you're teaching this new nurse. As you know, nursing school is tough and that first year of nursing is even tougher. It is essential for their development that you create an environment in which they feel safe asking you even the most basic and simple questions. Even if it's something you think they should know, do not use that opportunity to belittle them. That will send a message loud and clear: "Do not come to me for a question unless absolutely necessary. Pretend you know the answers so I don't make you look stupid."

This is dangerous. This fosters silence in health care, where nurses don't speak up when they don't know the right way to do something. This is a big problem in the field of nursing. There are so many nurses who pretend they know things that they actually don't—and patients suffer because of it.

You are your orientee's source of knowledge; you are whom they go to for questions. Foster an environment in which they feel safe talking to you. Be understanding; be nice. However, if your orientee is asking many basic questions that cause you to question if they are appropriate for this job, that's a different situation and needs to be handled differently. We will talk about that more later.

Goal Setting for Results

It is essential that you set attainable, measureable goals for every shift, starting day one. Creating appropriate goals was always a challenge for me. It took some time to consider all of the necessary factors when deciding upon a goal.

A helpful way to remember and structure these is the SMART goals mnemonic:

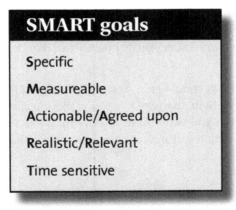

SMART goals

Specific

Measureable

Actionable/Agreed upon

Realistic/Relevant

Time sensitive

Creating appropriate goals is especially essential for new graduate nurses. The more you get to know them and their skill level, the easier it will be to identify goals. Goal setting facilitates progression. You want them to get through orientation as quickly as possible without any lulls. I recommend starting each shift with a short two-minute pep talk going over your goals with them so they know where to focus. They learn so much at the beginning, it can be really helpful to know where to focus and when. As orientation progresses, your goals will become more complex.

Some examples for goals starting day one can be: familiarize yourself with our phone system and take initiative to answer phones if sitting at the desk; know how to operate the medication dispensing machine independently; be able to hook patient up to bedside monitor (or telemetry

Sample Weekly Orientation/Documentation Sheet

Nursing Orientation—St. Francis Medical Center, Intensive Care Unit

Name: _____ Preceptor(s): _____

Week of orientation: _____ Dates: _____ Shift(s): _____

This week's goals	1. _____
	2. _____
	3. _____
Next week's goals	1. _____
	2. _____
	3. _____

Orientation Weekly Experience Summary

Patient Types	Specific Deficits
Lines/Drains/Airways	Special Monitoring
Procedures/Technical Skills/Tasks	Policies and Procedures Reviewed
Specific Medications Discussed	Time and Problem Management
Documentation	Delegation

Goals, Comments, Recommendations

Goals Met	Goals Not Met and Explanation
Praise, Constructive Criticism	Additional Experience Needed

Preceptee's signature: _____ Date: _____

Preceptor's signature: _____ Date: _____

box) independently; be able to verbalize the setup for the room for an incoming admission; know where all essential supplies and rooms are located, and so forth.

Documentation for Orientation

It's important to keep a detailed record of what you have gone over with them (specific policies and procedures), as well as what kinds of patients you have cared for and various skills that have been checked off. Many hospitals have a form they require for documentation of orientation progression; however, not all do. These documentation forms include information such as the week of orientation, the patients they have cared for, the policies they've reviewed, procedures they have completed, specific goals, opportunities for improvement, and praise. Each week, you review this with them, and you both sign it. You keep a copy and they get a copy (and so does the manager, if required).

This may sound like a lot of work and indeed it can be a bit tedious. However, this documentation (whether or not your hospital requires it) is essential. Over time, the days blend into each other, and you will forget the things they have done. Heaven forbid you get to a point where they are not progressing and they claim you never educated them about specific things. That is when you go back to your records and say, "We actually did discuss this during week four, and you signed that you did in fact have experience with this particular policy."

I have included a sample documentation sheet sample that a colleague, Melissa Stafford, BSN RN CCRN SCRN, developed. (She is also one of the best preceptors I have ever observed.) It can be adapted to fit the needs of your unit. I recommend having an electronic copy of whichever documentation tool you will use and then fill it out continually through each week. As soon as they start to become more independent and need you to become more hands-off, you'll have more time to fill this out during each shift rather than after each week or shift.

Identifying a Mentor

As important as it is to start up the documentation—needed to track and record your orientee's progression throughout her or his orientation—it is just as essential to establish both a mentor and a preceptor. More about mentoring in Chapter 4.

I like to compare these two relationships to athletics. The preceptor is similar to the head coach and the preceptee is the athlete. Sometimes the head coach is nice, sometimes they are motivating, and sometimes they must hold people accountable and have tough conversations. However, that is how the effective preceptor–preceptee relationship should look. At the end of the day, it is the preceptor's responsibility to make sure the preceptee is a safe and competent nurse, much like it is the coach's responsibility to make their players successful athletes.

While a preceptor–orientee relationship is similar to and head coach–athlete relationship, a mentor–orientee relationship is similar to an assistant coach–athlete relationship. An assistant coach is more of a motivator and encourager. Someone who the athlete can confide in, get some support, and understand some of the dynamics of the team as well as the personality of the head coach. Most importantly, the assistant coach is someone the athlete can trust. They trust the assistant coach's judgment, and they trust that their concerns and feelings are kept confidential. This is why having both a preceptor and a mentor is essential in the successful development of an orientee. I will discuss this much more in depth in the next chapter.

Time Management: Drowning a Little

While they're figuring out their own time management in Phases Two and Three of orientation (more details to come starting on page 36), I generally let them get a little overwhelmed. Here's why.

This way they can see and feel that maybe that wasn't the best way to organize their time in those situations or maybe they should have prioritized differently. They will remember it better because they went through it and felt how inefficient it was. This is much more effective than telling them what to do, in what order, at the beginning of the day. They will not develop their own ability to prioritize and manage their time if you always tell them what to do. They will become dependent on others and not develop confidence in their own skills.

When I touch base with them, I talk about things I observed that could have been done more efficiently to save them some time. I also look at how they prioritize their tasks and if there's any room for improvement. Remember, the tendency is to do things that they know how to do first, not necessarily the things that are the priority. For example, if they need to hang a unit of blood or go give scheduled PO meds, they'll probably head to give the meds first. Redirect them as needed.

It's important to empower them to take responsibility for their patient load as soon as possible. The scariest part of being out of orientation is knowing that you are ultimately responsible for your patient's well-being without anyone checking behind you. The earlier you can empower them to take responsibility for their patients, the better. When giving and getting the report, make sure the off-going nurse is giving the report to your orientee and not you. Make sure they're paging the physicians and rounding with them. Whenever anyone asks any questions about the patient, refer them to your orientee. At this point, you're in the background to help PRN and to double check behind charting and task completion.

Furthermore, praise is extremely important in all of these phases. It is really scary and humbling to be a brand new nurse or an experienced nurse switching specialties. They're constantly being told they're wrong. So when they do something well or right, make sure they know it. It can go a long, long way.

Your Progression as Preceptor

One thing that you do not want to forget to assess at least weekly is your personal progression as the preceptor. Everyone learns differently, and if you are not catering to your orientee's learning style, they may not be getting all they could be out of orientation. Information can be lost in translation. You need to find out from your orientee if you're doing a good job. Some people need their preceptor to back off earlier than others, some need more hands-on teaching for a longer period of time, some need a lot of positivity, and some do not. You never know what your preceptee needs if you do not ask. It is really difficult for a brand new person on a unit to tell one of the informal leaders (i.e., you) to stop rounding with physicians for them, or answering all of their phone calls, or doing things they are able to do. That conversation is really hard to initiate. Therefore, you as the leader and preceptor need to make sure you ask. And please, be prepared for the answer. It may not all be positive; they may have some needs that are not being met. Please do not take it personally. The priority is to get this person to be a functional, efficient, safe care provider and coworker for you and the rest of your team. While we want everyone to be kind and nice, we don't want people to be so concerned about being nice that they're not honest about their needs. So if they say something that is tough to hear, make sure you respond appropriately and professionally in the conversation and take some time to think about what they said.

I asked an orientee that question once, and I was so glad that she was so respectfully honest to me. She told me that I was being so positive every single shift that she had no idea she was doing anything wrong. Even when she would mess up, I would spin it in a positive way so it never really sunk in that it was not good. She was right. She was so, so right. I did a disservice to her by first of all not asking her this sooner in the orientation process, but also by not being totally honest with her about her progression. I didn't want to have these tough conversations, I didn't want to be "grumpy old Kati preceptor, telling someone they were doing something wrong," but it is essential that preceptors do that! So what if they think you're a jerk? If you're instilling good, efficient, safe habits into this person, they will thank you later.

I'd like to give you an example of the scenario where the preceptor seemed like a jerk in orientation, but the preceptee ended up being thankful later on. One of my coworkers told me about her orientation process and how frustrated she was every single day by this one nurse who kept harping on her about her alarms. The second one of her patient's alarms were going on, the nurse was on her to address this. She said it was incredibly frustrating and annoying every single day of her 12-week orientation. However, now she is so thankful that she was on her for her alarms because it is engrained in her to answer them quickly. I am pretty thankful for this nurse too, because she does this with all new nurses on our unit and we do not suffer from alarm fatigue.

Communication and Challenges

Another essential aspect of goal setting, achievement, and progression with your orientee is communicating with your coworkers. If you are working on getting your orientee to be able to settle a new admission into the intensive care unit and want them to know all the things that need to be completed upon arrival, make sure your team knows not to just go in and do everything for them. They need to be challenged and pushed. In reality, most of the time they will not be left alone to deal with all of these issues because their coworkers will help them. However, we all know that does not always happen. Sometimes you're short-staffed; sometimes other patients are having an emergency as well, and suddenly they have to handle something independently that they've always had help with. We want them to be prepared for that scenario and empowered to handle it appropriately.

Additionally, as previously discussed, something I like to really infuse into the mentality of new hires is answering alarms in a timely fashion. Most of the time, the entire unit responds to various alarms, depending on who is at the desk or near the room. However, if you are in orientation on my unit, you answer all of your own alarms. This may be annoying and tedious, but it instills a sense of urgency from day one regarding answering your alarms in a timely fashion because you cannot always count on your coworker to take care of it. Therefore, if an alarm is going off on a patient of the orientee, all of the nurses on the unit know to ask the preceptor first if they are allowed to address the alarm for them. The entire team is aware that answering alarms quickly is the goal of every new hire, so they all know to ask first before addressing them. This also presents a good learning opportunity if they are continually addressing an unnecessary alarm whose settings should be changed. Alarm fatigue kills, and breaking the habit is harder than instilling good habits at the beginning.

This is why orientation should be tough. They need to go through the worst of it during orientation with a preceptor, so when they're out on their own they can handle it because they've done it before. Nurses on orientation should have a tough assignment every single shift. They should be working their butts off. When they get off orientation, it should feel easy to them. Being a former college athlete, I liken this process to athletics. You want to practice hard and be ready for anything, so that when game time comes, you are so prepared that handling the tough situations is like second nature. Orientation is practice; game time starts day one off orientation.

When you are precepting someone, make sure you're picking out the patients that they will be taking appropriately. You don't want to make them so overwhelmed they can't handle it, but you want it to be challenging. You want to look at giving them a tough, not impossible, assignment. Think about what would be challenging and select patients accordingly. Similarly, the other nurses on your unit should know and accept that the orientee gets first selection of patients because every single shift of their orientation counts. Sorry if your BFF coworker had those patients yesterday and really wants them back, but two of them are perfect for this orientee today and they will be taking them. There should not be any frustration or animosity. Growing your newbies effectively and efficiently is the foundation of a successful unit. Maybe your coworker loves taking care of tracheostomy patients or patients on an oscillator, but if your orientee needs experience with that, they will always have the priority. This attitude needs to be instilled in the entire unit. To do so, communicate respectfully and appropriately when selecting patients for your newbie to take.

Promote Independence

When you and your preceptee are taking care of patients, make sure that you are backing off and promoting independence as quickly as possible. If your orientee has five patients, they are responsible for five patients and must how to learn how to balance their time and tasks appropriately. It is not a situation in which they take three patients, you take two and you help them complete tasks continually throughout the shift.

If your orientee is really busy and you, as the primary nurse, would be calling the doctor, don't page for them. They need to learn to prioritize their time and balance their tasks. This can be tough when you have some a few patients who are not doing well or it gets busy. Know your limit. Don't let harm ever come to the patient, but always make sure you are hands-off when they progress to that point. This is absolutely essential; I cannot stress this enough. Honestly, by the last phase I will outline, you should be at the nurse's station most of the shift. You should be checking their charts, filling out paperwork, available to answer questions, and so on. You should not be hands-on with their patient care because they should be handling the majority of their shift independently.

This can be more challenging than some may realize. Sometimes it would be way easier and faster if you just took care of some things for them, but you are precepting them so they can learn. You are doing a disservice to them by enabling them. So what if they get overwhelmed or are behind? They need to learn during orientation how to handle this independently with you nearby for guidance; not lean on you every time they get busy to bail them out. They need to learn how to handle stressful situations during orientation.

When They're Not Progressing

Not every nurse is capable of working in every unit. Not everyone is cut out for critical care, the emergency department, labor and delivery, med–surg, dialysis, and so forth. Sometimes someone who looked great on paper and in the interview is not working out on the unit, and sometimes people think they know what it will be like to work on a specific unit but once they get there and see what it's really like, they are no longer interested. The goal is to do whatever you can to get the person to be successful on the unit, but it doesn't always happen.

When you, as the preceptor or even mentor, start to notice some red flags, make sure you document this appropriately. This is why those goal-setting sheets are absolutely essential. You're able to sit down and really look at everything you have discussed over the weeks. You can see what specific goals they had and why they did or did not meet them. Sometimes there are legitimate reasons why goals were not met. However, when this becomes a pattern, it is concerning.

If you are consistently communicating goals, having meetings regularly to talk about expectations and progression, and they are meeting with their mentor, they may be able to tell for themselves they're not a great fit for the unit before it's even necessary to say something. If they see that shift after shift, week after week, they're still coming up short even though they're trying their best, they may want to talk about their options with you and management. Again, that's okay. It's better to identify this now rather than six months in when they're totally overwhelmed, patients are suffering, and coworkers are not getting the support they need.

However, some people may just need a push in a different direction. Maybe they're not progressing because they need a different preceptor. Maybe their learning style is so vastly different from your teaching method that it would be best to switch things up. Or maybe they just need some more time on orientation with the heat turned up. Sometimes a nurse can seem like they're not going to fly, then you turn the heat on and they excel. Again, the key is consistent communication. Needs must be identified, expectations and goals must be clear, and the entire team needs to be aware of all of this.

| Phase 1.
The Lay of
the Land | Phase 2.
The Training
Wheels Are On | Phase 3.
Let Them Fly |

Phases of Orientation

I have been through multiple preceptor training courses, precepted new grads and experienced nurses, and observed many others get trained. Despite the location, facility, floor, preceptor, or preceptee, I have noticed that the process of orientation typically evolves in three separate phases. While the duration may vary depending on the aforementioned variables, the phases themselves are relatively standard. My hope is that by viewing the nursing orientation process in this structure, it will help guide you as you educate the new hires on your unit. Please keep in mind that below has been cultivated from my personal experience and the purpose is to present to you one way of looking at the process of orientation.

Phase One: The Lay of the Land
The first few shifts are utilized for observation. They need to see the flow and culture of the unit and patient population. The patients assigned to you are still your patients; however, your orientee is going to be given tasks to complete, all while getting familiar with the flow of the unit.

During patient care, have them perform simple tasks: draw up medications, calculate dosages, administer IV/subcutaneous medications, start IVs, put in feeding tubes, demonstrate appropriate documentation, insert Foley catheters, put patients on telemetry, or whatever are routine tasks for your unit.

When they ask how to do these things, show them how to look up policies and procedures. Doing so ensures that you are teaching them the correct way, because policies and procedures change routinely and what you were taught during your orientation may not reflect the current policy. I always learn so much each time I orient someone because inevitably some policy has changed between now and the last time I oriented someone.

You will find yourself asking, "What does the policy say?" over and over again, but you need to get them into that habit. During orientation, they have the time to look up more things than when they're out on their own. Instill this behavior in them. You want their instinct to be looking up the policy when they don't know how to do something, not just asking another nurse.

It's also important during this time to introduce them to everyone. And I mean, everyone! Introduce them to the housekeeper, the CNAs, fellow nurses, physicians, nurse practitioners, physician assistants, case managers, dieticians, and food service workers. This makes them feel like they're part of the team and assimilates them much more quickly. The sooner they feel like they're part of the team, the sooner they'll feel comfortable working independently.

During Phase One when you're showing them the ropes, demonstrate your awesome and efficient time-management skills and your routine for how you walk through your day. For example, I would show them how, after report, I look at my patients as a whole and decide whom I am going to see first and talk to them about how I came to that conclusion. Then I talk them through my thought process for deciding the order in which I will see the rest of my patients. Typically, during this time there will be many interruptions and reasons for the order you were going to see your patients to change, so explain this to them as you're reprioritizing your day. I also explain the other methods of time management I tried that failed, which further solidifies why I do what I do.

It is important to remember to give your orientee a consistent routine related to time management. Once they're out on their own, they can start to improvise and change how they manage their time. But right now they don't know what all of their options are, so they can't make an appropriate judgment on what they like best. This can be applicable even to experienced nurses who are starting on your unit. While they may have had a routine where they used to work, it may not be the most efficient and best way to tackle their day in this unit.

Something that expert nurses forget (because they're experts) is the "why" behind everything. The things we do become so normal and natural, we just don't have to think about the "why" anymore. Remember, these newbies need to know the why. This is important in their professional development into a safe care provider. Even if it seems menial, you must explain the why behind everything. Examples include: why it is essential to make sure a patient has voided after removing a Foley catheter, why you administer blood products more slowly to someone with congestive heart failure, or why you treat pain first before increasing sedation. The list goes on and on.

Another thing I like to do is find information for them to read at home about our specific patient population. Whether they're on orientation or not, families expect nurses to know the basics of the disease process that is affecting their loved ones. After nursing school, they know a little bit of everything. They don't necessarily know the complex details of the various surgeries the patients of this unit typically experience, the expected healing time, or typical discharge meds and side effects. Now is the time that you can get your newbie nurse to really focus on the specific things.

Checklist of Phase One To-Dos

- Formally introduce them to everyone they'll need to know: CNAs, MDs, PAs, NPs, transporters, and all who support the nursing team.

- Explain your time-management technique and why you do things in the order that you do them.

- Explain how you approach prioritization, which is ever-changing throughout the day.

- Demonstrate appropriate delegation as well as account-ability when tasks are delegated.

- Have them observe how you interact with patients and families, physicians, and support staff.

- Get them familiar with documentation.

- Have them take report right along with you so they can choose the report sheet they want to use and become familiar with it.

- Get them familiar with your IV pumps, tubing, and all of the other equipment and supplies.

- Find information specific to your patient population, print it off, and have them read about it at home. Quiz them on it the next day.

- Show them how to look up policies and procedures.

- Get them familiar with the house phone numbers and departments. Take them wherever you go in the hospital to show them around.

Depending on their progression, this can last two to three weeks before you move on.

Phase Two: The Training Wheels Are On

Phase Two begins with your orientee taking a patient on their own. You'll be able to tell they're ready for this by seeing how they're picking up what you're telling them. Sometimes, they'll tell you flat out.

During this phase, they take one patient (or more, if appropriate) on their own. After seeing how you take care of a patient, they should be able to adequately care for one person while you're nearby for questions.

They take and give report on their patient. They do everything for them, even call physicians and support staff, as needed. They complete all of the documentation. They talk to the patient and their patient's loved ones and provide education.

Again, if they don't know how to do something, always direct them to the policy first. With one (or only a few) patient(s), they should have time to go look up the policies for everything.

Continue to give them homework. Print off information about your patient population and quiz them the next day.

During this time, I start to ask all of my *why* questions. Depending on their progression and knowledge base, I try to challenge them with the questions. I also try to think of questions that patients may ask about their care plan.

- Why do you think they're on subcutaneous heparin?
- Why are they on Colace and Pepcid?
- Why do we need to do a bladder scan if they didn't void six hours after you removed the Foley?
- Why do you think you needed to put your patient with congestive heart failure on oxygen after he got two units of blood?
- Why do you think we need a central line when initiating vasoactive medications?
- Why is it imperative that you lay patients completely flat when removing their central venous catheter?
- Why are we still giving them IV pain medication when we have oral pain medication ordered?

Whenever they come to me with a question, I just ask it back to them to see what they think. I want them to develop their critical thinking skills. They need to go from being task-oriented to being big picture–oriented. While developing these skills, it's important to not give away the answers quickly.

Let them think. (This is much harder than it sounds! It is quite challenging for me not to give away answers.)

Additionally, if other members of the health care team ask them questions about the patient, don't immediately answer for them. Give them time to think and respond. This can also be quite challenging when you already know the answers to all of their questions and realize the person asking the questions is in a rush. Try your best to resist and interject only when necessary.

Remember, you want to encourage your orientee to ask questions. This is why it is important not to act like they're stupid if they get one wrong or do something incorrectly. Handle those situations with grace. Please don't use that opportunity to make someone feel bad about themselves. That's the terrible *nurses eating their young* thing.

It is really important during all phases of orientation that you are treating everyone around you with the utmost respect. If you are talking badly about other people in front of your orientee, they see and hear that. If you're not being respectful of the CNAs, you're telling them it's okay to do that. If you are nice to someone's face and once they leave, you talk about them, your orientee will start to wonder what you say about them. They are watching how you do everything, including how you interact with others. If you want them to be a good nurse, supportive coworker, and someone you can rely on, it is imperative that you model that yourself.

Phase Three: Let Them Fly
In critical care, whenever we remove a patient's breathing tube (or extubate them), we say we're going to "let them fly" and see how they do. We evaluate the likelihood of them being able to successfully breathe on their own, remove the tube, and watch them closely to see how they do before we move them out of critical care. You can never be 100% sure that they will succeed without the endotracheal tube, but at some point you must try. You can always reinsert the tube if needed.

That's exactly what the third phase should look like. We evaluate during the second phase of orientation if they are ready to take on their own patient load. Once we have seen them demonstrate skills that indicate this, we let them fly and see how they do while we are nearby for guidance and to facilitate their problem solving. We can always jump back in if needed, but the goal is for them to be working independently, coming to you for help less frequently as time progresses.

They should become more confident in completing tasks and start to think more and more about the big picture. They should be able to anticipate obstacles. They should be figuring out their time management style. They should be appropriately discussing the plan of care with other members of the health care team. They should be delegating properly.

I have a little conference at the beginning of the shift right after report and outline our goals for the day. When deciding on goals, I think about the things they are struggling with and make those the priority.

Example:

> *Alright, today starts week seven and we have a few goals today. First, I want you to make sure you're acknowledging new orders that come through within one hour of them being placed. Our second goal will be to give all medications on time unless extenuating circumstances present themselves. And our final goal is to delegate appropriately all day today so that you are working at the top of your license consistently. At 1100, I will check your charting. At 1500, we'll see where we are with our goals and what we can do or change to ensure we're on track to meet them. If you encounter any roadblocks, please come ask me. However, I want you to try to be as independent as possible.*

As these nurses on orientation become more confident in themselves and work independently, they may have even more questions than before, but they will be at a higher level. They will be developing their critical thinking skills, starting to figure out what to question, and so on. Questions are good, but most of the time they know the answer already and they're just checking to make sure they have acted appropriately. This is great, but you want promote reliance on their own knowledge, not dependence on their coworkers. If you always give them the answer every time, they will only keep coming to you with more questions.

Whenever they come up to me to ask a question, I basically ask the question back to them to see what their thought process is. Essentially, I provide a response that says, "Okay, so the situation you described is _____. What do you think is the best way to handle this?" Nine times out of ten, they give you the right answer. If they give you the wrong answer, they have also told you their thought process, and you can correct that as well. Orientees crave reassurance. While it is important to reassure them, you don't want them to become dependent on you telling them what to do. Reassure and praise them when they do a good job, when they handle a tough situation well, when they educate a patient well, and so on. That's the avenue reassurance should come from, not every time they have a question about something you know they know the answer to.

Precepting is a lot of work, especially at the beginning. You really have to be on top of your game with each shift, teaching, encouraging, and holding them accountable. If done successfully, after orientation is over not only will you will be left with a strong, confident, and safe colleague, but you will also have found that you have grown as a nurse yourself.

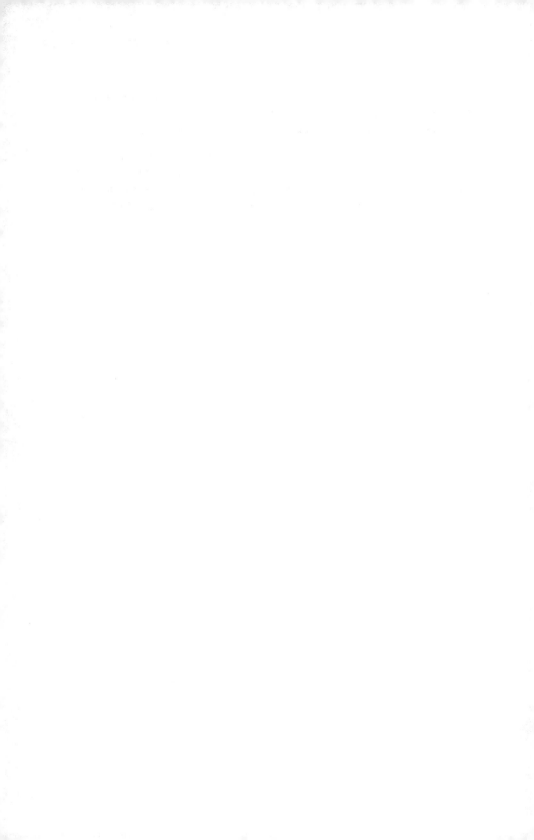

4

Mentoring New Nurses: Growing the Newbies

Mentoring and precepting are very different ways of developing new nurses. However, people tend to look at them as one and the same. Both roles are essential in the development of new employees, and appropriate mentorship benefits more than just the newbies.

Mentoring is another aspect of professional development for advanced beginners and competent nurses. As you will see, it differs from precepting and can offer different challenges and rewards. Just like precepting, you don't have to be a nurse with decades of experience to help grow and develop new nurses. Advanced beginners and competent nurses more recently went through all of the challenges of becoming a nurse and can relate to their new coworker more easily, as all of those thoughts, feelings, and emotions are still fresh. While the mentor–mentee relationship is not quite as formal as the preceptor–preceptee relationship, there should still be some structure involved. First, I'll go over why mentoring works, then I'll further differentiate between mentoring and precepting, followed by some practical advice, and finally an example of a mentor–mentee relationship during a 12-week orientation.

Appropriate Mentoring Works on Multiple Levels

According to the 2015 National Healthcare Retention and RN Staffing Report, the current national average turnover rate for bedside RNs is 17.2%. This is up from 16.4% in 2014 and from 11.2% in 2011. The highest turnover rates were in medical–surgical, behavioral health, and emergency departments, while the lowest turnover rates were noted in pediatrics and women's health (Nursing Solutions, Inc., 2016, p. 1).

The cost of turnover is astronomical. With hospital budgets being cut to keep up with the dwindling reimbursement from the federal government, the money lost when nurses leave is literally walking out the door. According to this same report, "The average cost of turnover for a bedside RN ranges from $37,700 to $58,400" (Nursing Solutions, Inc., 2016, p. 1). Meaning, when a bedside RN leaves a hospital, it can cost them anywhere within that range for that one nurse walking away (related to costs from training them, overtime pay and floating nurse pay to make up for deficit, and other avenues of lost revenue from that RN leaving). This results "in the average hospital losing $5,200,000 to $8,100,000" when you figure in all of the nurses that leave within that year (Nursing Solutions, Inc., 2016, p. 1). Furthermore, every percentage change in nursing turnover can either save or cost the facility $373,200 (Nursing Solutions, Inc., 2016, p. 1). Unhappy nurses mean major costs for hospitals that are frequently unseen.

Nursing turnover is a big deal. It will continue to be a focal point for cost savings for years to come if people do not fully embrace or recognize its importance.

What does this have to do with mentoring, you ask? Successful nursing mentorship programs can profoundly impact nursing retention. For example, according to Fox (2010), in 2004 St. Francis Hospital and Health Centers saw their first-year nursing turnover rates increase significantly. They decided to implement a formal mentorship program with the goals of increasing satisfaction and decreasing turnover. After a one-year pilot study, the pilot group's turnover rate went from 31% (well above the national average) to 0%. In 2009, the centers' overall turnover rate sat well below the national average at 10.3% (Fox, 2010, p. 311).

These numbers are staggering. If it costs on average $379,500 today for each percentage change in turnover rates, and this hospital's average went from 31% to 10.3%, they could have roughly saved over $7.8 million in 2015 on nursing retention alone. This does not even factor in the impact this had on patient satisfaction and outcomes, but one can only imagine.

It makes sense, right? If someone is invested in your development as a bedside nurse practically, and another person is also invested in your values, builds a relationship with you, and guides you through the overwhelming processes of embarking on this journey, you are more inclined to stay. It saves you stress and the hospital significant amounts of money, and, according to Gelinas & Bohlen (2002), the patients have better outcomes.

Now that we have explored the profound benefits of mentoring, let's dig deeper into the difference between a nursing mentor and a nursing preceptor.

The Nurse Preceptor

Many nurses are very comfortable with the definition of a preceptor, as many have functioned in this role at some point in their career. The preceptor is ultimately responsible for the new nurse's orientation. They are responsible for the orientee's education and development, and all day-to-day activities during orientation. They are directly supervising the new nurse. Preceptors complete formal evaluations, discuss progress (or lack thereof), set goals, provide constructive criticism, and many other things. This is a formal relationship with very defined expectations. Preceptors may spend time trying to facilitate and encourage the new nurse's relationships with the nursing staff and other members of the health care team, but it is neither the priority nor the focus.

While it is absolutely necessary to have a preceptor, having this person as the new employee's only source of support during this transition can be detrimental. While the new nurse is busy learning the technical side of their new role, they are left lacking in emotional support, encouragement, and different perspectives, all while dealing with increasing anxiety attempting to meet all of the preceptor's expectations. Naturally, this can become very overwhelming very quickly.

The Nurse Mentor

Mentors have a very different function and purpose. They are not there to directly supervise or provide evaluations. They do not oversee the new nurse's day-to-day activities. According to McKinley's (2004) article in the AACN's journal, *Clinical Issues*, "Mentoring focuses on the human connection between the experienced and novice nurse and serves as a special way to transfer knowledge." She continues: "Effective mentoring demonstrates proactive leadership and fosters leadership development by focusing beyond processes and skills to value and culture" (p. 206). So, the preceptor focuses on skill, while the mentor focuses on value and culture. While very different, both are absolutely essential in the successful development and assimilation of the new nurse.

Therefore, you as the mentor are there to develop a trusting relationship with the new nurse. You are their go-to person for things outside the technical teaching of becoming a successful bedside nurse. You are they go to when they need to ask, "So, Dr. Alfonso was really rude to me on the phone today. He asked me all of these questions, and I didn't know the answers and got flustered. What do I do?"

You can reply, "The thing you have to know about Dr. Alfonso, and many other physicians, is that if you call them with a concern, they expect you to be able to answer a lot of questions about that patient. You don't just want to rattle off your question for them because they'll probably have at least five back for you. Make sure you know your vitals, labs, meds, all of that, before calling. He can be kind of rude about it, just make sure you're standing up for yourself when you speak to him and try not to take it personally. He is a pretty nice guy overall but can be short with people if they're not prepared. Seriously, you're doing fine, and he's done that to many people before." You can educate them on the culture of the unit and provide support after a frustrating situation.

While the preceptor may tell the new nurse to call the doctor and help them implement the orders received, the mentor can help them troubleshoot developing interpersonal relationships with the entire health care team. This can include telling them everyone's nuances, habits, personality traits, and quirks. If one nurse on the next shift prefers report to be as detailed as possible and the next nurse prefers it to be as concise as possible, it's helpful to know and understand those things prior.

The Team Approach to Precepting and Mentoring

Being a new nurse on a unit is extremely overwhelming. There is a large amount of information they are responsible for knowing quickly. The preceptor is constantly providing new information. It can feel like they're trying to get a sip of water from a fire hose. As expert nurses, it can be easy to forget how completely overwhelming those first six months on the job really were. We get so acclimated into our roles and so used to our day to day that we forget that at one time we had to be taught how to complete every single task we now do without thinking about.

Newbies are trying as hard as they can to absorb as much information as possible from this one person. Therefore, it can beneficial for a completely different person to provide additional encouragement, support, information, and inspiration. The new nurse is constantly just trying not to screw up, trying not to get corrected, trying to do their best. The preceptor is there guiding them through that and will correct them when needed and praise them when needed. However, the mentor can help them process various situations, circumstances, and relationships objectively and outside of the relationship with the preceptor.

If they, as a new nurse, are being corrected and educated frequently, the relationship can easily become strained and the feelings of anxiety and being overwhelmed can quickly become unbearable. People can become frustrated, mad, upset, or discouraged when going through this process. However, if they have a mentor to process situations with whom they can trust, it can put things into perspective. This mentor understands the new nurse's values and has taken the time to develop an interpersonal relationship with them, outside of teaching the ins and outs of a unit. This mentor can marry the two distinct sides of nursing on that particular unit: the technical, skill-related side of nursing, and the interpersonal, cultural, communication, and value-related side of nursing. The foundation of a successful nurse is built upon a balance of both. Nurses cannot meet the needs of patients, coworkers, and self if they are too focused on the technical side or too focused on the cultural, value-based side. Both need to be appropriately encouraged, developed, and enhanced. This is why it is essential that both preceptor and mentor are heavily invested in their respective responsibilities to this new nurse.

Who Should Be a Mentor?

Mentors should be people on the unit that others respect. They are good nurses who care for their patients holistically. They know how to work some of the more complicated equipment and be the calm in the chaos, but also know when to stop and be with a patient when they're having a tough emotional moment.

They are the informal leaders to whom others go to for advice, related to both patient care and the bigger picture of nursing. They are honest, trustworthy, respectful people. They do not necessarily have to have the most education or most certifications, or be a part of the most professional organizations (although that's fantastic if they are!), but they value providing optimal patient care based on evidence-based practice. These are not the people who roll their eyes at change. They are the people who openly embrace and accept change. They provide solutions, they do not add to the problem. They are good role models. They do not engage in gossip, they empower and encourage others. They are someone that you see on the schedule and are relieved to see they are working with you today.

Mentor Responsibilities and Expectations

The role of the mentor is somewhat less concrete than the role of the preceptor. Things the mentor is responsible for can include, but are not limited to, the items in the following table.

Responsibility	Example
Navigate the culture and flow of the hospital outside of nursing-related tasks	Show them how to contact the timekeeper or payroll. Take them to everyone's favorite coffee kiosk. Introduce them to various people, like the nursing directors, security officers, transport staff, all of those whose work touches on nursing care.
Encourage	Send them a text message or call them after a particularly challenging shift to see how they're doing and offer some encouragement.
Coach	Prepare them mentally for an upcoming challenge, like taking a full patient load for the first time or their first day off orientation. Provide encouragement and strategies for success, and follow up to see how it went.
Develop a relationship	Get to know the new nurse on a personal level. Learn and appreciate their values and personal culture. Show that you care about how they are doing. Continually check in and figure out the best way to support them. Meet outside of work, ask how life outside of this new job is going, and offer support and bonding.
Maintain confidentiality	Initially inform them that their conversations are always going to be confidential and private, and make sure to faithfully maintain this and not discuss anything with others.
Encourage professional growth	Show them the various resources, committees, and groups at the hospital to become more involved. Introduce them to the leaders of these groups. Make sure their name is known around the hospital. Provide them with information on getting reimbursed for being affiliated with professional organizations, shared governance, the process for tuition reimbursement if they want to go back to school, how to start a research project, and other professional development particulars.

Leading by Example

Something to be conscious of as you are mentoring someone is your demeanor and attitude as a coworker. The ultimate goal is for this person to be a successful, competent nurse and coworker to you and the rest of the team. You want this person to turn into someone you trust and rely upon, who will be part of the team for years to come.

Therefore, if you, in your personal interactions with your mentee, are sincere and supporting, but you talk about how ridiculous the float nurse was who didn't even know how to draw labs off an arterial line when you're sitting at the nurse's station with a bunch of coworkers, they will notice. They, like any other person, will wonder what you say about them when they are not around.

Observing this behavior from a mentor may hit them harder and on a more personal level than if they observed it from their preceptor. I say this because your mentee may confide really personal things to you that they do not share with their preceptor, which can include personal struggles with the preceptor and other staff members. You want to encourage them to feel comfortable coming to you with these concerns so you can help them navigate these relationships. This is why maintaining confidentiality is an essential piece of the relationship. You want your mentee to feel comfortable and confident that they can come to you with their embarrassing concerns, mistakes, and situations and know you will not use that vulnerability as an opportunity to make fun of them or tell others.

So, if you are openly discussing the inadequacy of others, it may cause your mentee to question themselves, feel insecure, and withdraw from their relationship with you. If this continues, it will leave the new nurse feeling isolated, insecure, and unsupported throughout the process and beyond, thus defeating the mentoring process itself.

Know Your Boundaries

Inversely, it is important to remember that you are not there to solve the problems of your mentee. You are there to facilitate and encourage their independent problem solving and critical thinking. They may want to come to you to solve their problems. Respond with open-ended questions, facilitating their ability to handle it independently.

Furthermore, the tendency of the mentor can be to continually encourage their mentee. This is an essential function of the mentor; however, it should not be a constant and consistent response. This newbie needs to earn praise. Over-praising a mentee can lead them to believe it's insincere and look for affirmation from others they believe will be honest with them. This can damage the trusting relationship that was developed.

Over-praising a mentee can also prevent them from seeing the severity of various errors. If they are constantly reassured, even if they have committed a serious error or are developing poor skills, it will leave them unable to see the error of their ways. The continual praise clouds their ability to see what their needs really are, which, again, is a disservice to them. Honesty and balance is key.

When the Mentee Isn't as Awesome as They Seemed

However, we do know that sometimes your mentee may not come to you with legitimate concerns about others and how they can better themselves within their relationships, and instead just want to gossip. It is essential not to perpetuate this behavior. If they are not a new nurse but new to your unit, this may have been the culture for them in their last place of employment. Some people, as previously stated, use this as a survival tactic. Please nip it in the bud. It will create animosity, cliques, and isolation for others. It has been said many times that people quickly create bonds when they find common interests. Do not allow this common interest to be making fun of others, talking negatively, or gossiping.

Speaking as a bedside nurse, I do not like working with people who enjoy this. It is exhausting to be around and honestly embarrassing to be associated with. We are esteemed health care professionals, and if the last nurse left you with 20 things you need to clean up after and you spend the next 12 hours complaining to the your coworkers, you are not doing anyone any favors. It's not fun to listen to and does not take care of your problem. It just gives people not only a bad impression of that person but also of you for talking about it instead of speaking to the person.

Therefore, if your newbie nurse starts to engage in this behavior, do not tolerate it. Sometimes it is appropriate to say something to the effect of, "We don't really talk about each other on this unit. Usually if someone has a problem, they just bring it right to the person. Everyone is pretty responsive and respectful here, so it's no big deal if you really feel like that to just go tell them." Another way would be, "Look, I know you're new here to this unit, and I just want to let you know that if you have issues with people it's okay to just go them about it. Everyone here is pretty honest and would prefer if you just brought stuff to them directly. Then it doesn't turn into gossip. Everyone is pretty cool here." They may respond with a meek "Okay," followed by an awkward silence, but this sends a clear and powerful message early on in their career. Make sure you follow up on this conversation by not treating them differently. Calm and honest correction is not meant to be punitive, but it sure can feel that way regardless of how respectful and nice it was, so make sure you still approach them with the same enthusiasm as before, continuing to invest into your relationship.

Unfortunately, this is not always appropriate or the best way to handle this. Rarely are these big, sweeping, overtly mean comments. It is typically subtle rude things over time, which can be addressed gently and consistently. If they start to say something negative or gossip, you can always come back and say something positive about that person, or say, "Man, I hope people don't talk about me or you like that when we're not around," or just don't respond. If you do not respond or always respond in a way that diverts the conversation, they will stop coming to you with this negativity.

Sample Timeline of a Mentee–Mentor Relationship (12-Week Orientation)

When you are so rooted in the culture of a unit, it is really easy to forget how scary it can be when you're new. Nursing units are very close-knit cultures. The new people can feel like unwanted and uncomfortable outcasts until they have established themselves. This makes the orientation and acclimation process more difficult. However, if you can be more sensitive to this transition, I believe that your new nurses will become more confident in their skills and care earlier, allowing them to be better and more reliable coworkers sooner.

Some facilities have formal mentorship programs and some do not. Rest assured, you can provide this support to a new nurse without having a formal program in place.

Prior to the establishment of this relationship, ground rules need to be developed. This can be done between the preceptor, mentor, and manager. These ground rules can include a statement of confidentiality, a commitment to not gossip, an agreed-upon schedule of times to meet and check in both during and outside of work, as well as an attempt to ensure the mentor and mentee are working during some of the same shifts regularly.

Weeks 1 to 2: Getting Oriented to the Orientation

You are selected as their mentor with the consultation of the manager, preceptor, and mentee. You connect with the mentee and exchange contact information. A "get to know you" meeting outside of work or after an orientation day is a great idea. Get to know them, their values, who they are outside of nursing, why they decided to become a nurse, and what is really important to them. This will enable you to better support them throughout the process. Additionally, you can share similar information about yourself, so they begin to feel like they already know someone on the unit well. If you feel comfortable, connect with them on social media and via call or text to see how the first few days went.

Try to find common interests and maybe even work in a little inside joke or two. Getting an inside joke going between two people can immediately make someone feel more welcome, at home, and assimilated into the unit. This communicates that you care about them and your relationship and quickly facilitates the development of trust. You, as their mentor, want them to trust you. You want them to feel comfortable coming to you with any concerns so that you can encourage, reassure, troubleshoot, or direct them appropriately.

You can bring them coffee or just check in with them throughout the shifts. Observe the preceptor–preceptee relationship from afar; this will enable you to assess how you can best support them throughout orientation. For example, if you notice the preceptor is stern or very straightforward, reassure them, "Just so you know, she's not being mean so don't take her lack of warmth personally. It's her way of establishing a professional relationship and assessing your skills. She's all business at the beginning." A simple, supportive sentence like that can make a world of difference to a new nurse on their first week. It can prevent them from unnecessarily reading into situations that evoke feelings of insecurity and doubt.

Weeks 2 to 4: Building a Stronger and Trusting Relationship

You may get lunch or drinks outside of work to further root the relationship and invest in them. This continues to build trust and solidify the relationship. Even if schedules don't work out, just the simple gesture of trying to meet outside of work can mean a lot to a person in a totally new environment, new nurse or not. Do not underestimate the power of simple gestures.

Check-in with the preceptor and see if there's anything they're struggling with in particular. Many times, there may be something that the preceptor has explained or talked about multiple times that the new nurse just isn't getting right or that's not clicking in their head yet. The mentor can see if there's anything like this going on and decide how they can best support. Sometimes, the new nurse just needs it explained in a different way, or they need someone who's not a preceptor, whom they trust, to slowly walk through the task or concept with them.

I remember during my orientation into the neurosciences intensive care unit, I was trying to understand the differences between a subdural hematoma, intracerebral hematoma, epidural hematoma, intraventricular hemorrhage, and all of the various nursing considerations for each one. I had heard it a few times from my preceptor, and I still didn't get it. It finally clicked when someone else slowly took some time after a shift. For whatever reason, I just had to hear it explained differently, and suddenly I understood.

Also, keep in mind that your new nurse wants to impress their preceptor. They want to prove to them that they can handle this. They will put their best face forward for them. While this is great, it prevents the preceptor from being able to appropriately assess their needs.

I liken this to being new in a relationship. You show your best, most confident self to this new person and only after time do you feel comfortable being honest about your vulnerabilities and insecurities. This may be months down the line when this person gets to know the real you, after you have established trust. So, who do you go to when you have questions or concerns? Definitely not that new person! You go to your close friends or even family—the people you trust.

You, as the mentor, are like their close friends or family. The preceptor is like the new person they're in a relationship with. They're constantly trying to be the best, do their best, and impress them with what they know. With you, they should be comfortable being completely honest about the concerns, questions, or mistakes that they don't feel comfortable telling their preceptor. If they are open and honest with someone about their needs, these concerns will be much better addressed, they will be supported, and they will acclimate to your unit more quickly. They will be safer care providers because they are honest about what they don't know so appropriate education can be provided. Silence in health care is deadly.

We cannot engrain this behavior into a brand new nurse because it is very difficult to undo.

Again, trust is essential. Do not tell others what they share with you. They are sharing with you things they are vulnerable about and their insecurities. Facilitating this looks different for different people. To encourage open communication, be honest with them about your first experiences on the unit or times you made mistakes. If they called the wrong doctor and got yelled at, tell them a story of when something similar occurred and reassure them that it's okay. Casually bringing these things up when they're being honest with you can be more reassuring than you realize. Feel free to sing Michael Jackson's "You Are Not Alone" to them to really let them know that they are not the only person to experience this. That can be more reassuring and provide much more encouragement that you realize.

Weeks 4 to 6: Continuing to Invest
It's about the halfway point, and they should be getting more independent from their preceptor, more comfortable in the unit, and therefore, more comfortable exploring things outside of the unit. If you're going to the cafeteria, the blood bank, employee health, and the like, have them tag along to expose them to different areas of the hospital. Introduce them to people. Between the mentor and the preceptor introducing them to staff, they should be getting to know a large amount of people quickly and feel more at home.

Use these short trips to see how they're doing. See what competencies they've taken care of and what was tough for them, then tell them your tips and tricks for various things. Offer praise when they have accomplished goals, and provide strategies and support to enable them to tackle the obstacles that are more challenging or things they're nervous about.

If this nurse is new to nursing or brand new to your specialty, don't take for granted some of the daily tasks that they may never have seen performed before. For example, I work in a neurosciences intensive care unit, and we remove ventriculostomy drains from patient's skulls and place sutures. It's a pretty normal procedure for us because we do it so frequently; however, if you were a mentor in that situation and a patient of yours needed a drain removed, bring the newbie in and have them watch. Explain what you're doing, or have them perform the skill with your support. It can be refreshing and invigorating to complete new skills with a new person other than a preceptor. Someone else taking time to invest in showing someone something can just make them feel really good. They've accomplished a goal and someone was interested in them and thinking of them enough to include them and took the time to explain it to make sure they understood.

Weeks 6 to 10: Making Sure All Bases Are Covered

At this point of orientation, they should start to feel more a part of the team and less overwhelmed with some of the simpler things. Continue to text or call and check in. This can be a good time to see how they are doing with things that were not a priority at the start of orientation. Do they feel comfortable checking their email? Do they know what some of your sister units are, and where they would typically float? Have they met some of the informal leaders on those units? Are they comfortable with the entire scheduling and timekeeping process? Do they need to complete education or certification classes, and do they know how to sign up for them?

When I was first hired at both of the hospitals I have had the privilege of working at, I was given courses on my email and all of the above information during my orientation. However, I was on information overload. That information did not stick. I had so many questions about our timekeeping software, our educational requirements, our various resources related to human resources, and other issues that weren't directly related patient care. During the beginning of orientation, it went in one ear and out the other. It was only when I felt like I had my head above water a few weeks later that I went back to trying to understand and master these essential things.

While the preceptor may have gone over these things, it's good to have someone else checking in to make sure everything is in order. It may have gone in one ear and out the other, or, since it's not a priority, it may have been completely forgotten.

Furthermore, if you are involved in professional organizations, shared governance, or various committees, see if you can bring them along for a meeting or two. This will build your relationship further and encourage professional development. Insurmountable and scary tasks or commitments suddenly seem possible when you see someone else take part and do so with joy.

Also, make sure to check in with them regarding their relationship with the preceptor to make sure their needs are being met, their questions are being answered, and they are learning how to become an independently functioning nurse on your unit.

Weeks 10 to 12: Winding Down the Orientation

Their orientation is almost done! Woo-hoo!

This can create feelings of anxiety for the nurse because they will be leaving the safety net of their preceptor checking behind their work and supporting them. Treat the end of the orientation as an exciting time. Reassure them that they will be supported after orientation, and treat it as a positive and encouraging transition.

Ask them if they have specific concerns and see if you can address them specifically to enable them to be as confident as possible after the orientation is complete. If there are legitimate concerns about needing to extend orientation, it needs to be identified at this time. If so, a plan can be developed between the preceptor, mentor, and management team to ensure that a successful orientation extension with a very specific timeline that addresses the trainee's needs is established.

Celebrate their last day of orientation! Bring in a treat for them, and celebrate with the unit, which facilitates a team mentality. See if you can align your schedule so that you are also working with them on their very first day off orientation. Make sure they know that you are there to support them but that it's great and exciting that they're on their own. You don't want to provide a false sense of security because you want to promote independence.

After Orientation: Keep on Building Confidence

Continue to check in with them, invite them to unit activities, and consult them for their opinion on various things during your shift. We all, experienced or not, have questions every day. If people can confidently consult with a newer nurse on various things, it can really build the newer nurse's confidence and make them feel like a part of the team. If you only go to the one nurse who's been there for 23 years, but everyone else is completely capable of answering your question, it presents a very polarizing attitude. It tells people that you have to have decades of experience to be a good resource, which is not true. Many times, the newer nurses are more versed in the latest policies and procedures and are perfectly capable of being consulted with various nursing-related questions. So make sure you go to your newbie.

As you can tell, being a nurse mentor is a challenging but extremely rewarding role. The more you invest in the development of your coworkers, the more satisfied the staff will be and the more reliable your team will become.

5

Continuing Your Education: Going Back to School

After a certain point you may decide you want to look into going back to school. Nursing has so many wonderful and different options for continuing education, but it can be quite confusing. Let's discuss some of your various options, from a bachelor's degree all the way to a doctorate degree.

Bachelor of Science in Nursing (BSN)

In 2010, the Institute of Medicine issued a call to action for the profession of nursing: 80% of the nursing workforce should be BSN-prepared by 2020 (IOM, 2010). This can be a heated topic among nurses, as there are many associate's- and diploma-prepared nurses out there taking amazing and safe care of their patients. However, I do want to describe and outline why this initiative is so important for not only our profession but also our patients. I will do so by exploring the top four things I hear from people when discussing the associate's degree in nursing ADN versus BSN argument.

Nurses with a bachelor's degree are no different than nurses with an associate's degree. We all take and pass the same exam.

ADN nurses are more clinically prepared when they graduate from school. BSN graduates don't even know the basics.

ADN nurses can lead the health care team with an associate's degree.

All BSN programs do is force people to write more papers; it's not practical knowledge that helps our profession.

I have heard all of these things over and over in the hospital when this discussion comes up. I would like to clear the air once and for all on the BSN-versus-ADN nurse controversy. I will start by addressing each point I just mentioned.

"Nurses with a bachelor's degree are no different than nurses with an associate's. We all take and pass the same exam."

Response: Research shows that BSN-prepared nurses produce better outcomes. This is not someone's personal opinion or experience that demonstrates this fact; actual research (various studies over many years) continues to substantiate this. More BSN-prepared nurses equals fewer patient deaths. I cannot even begin to emphasize the importance of this.

In August 2014, a study posted in the *International Journal of Nursing Studies* stated that in South Korea and the University of Pennsylvania, a 9% drop in patient hospital deaths was noted with a 10% increase in BSN-prepared nurses (Cho et al., 2014).

Another article in the March 2013 issue of *Health Affairs* found that for every 10-point increase in percent of nurses with their BSN, there are an associated 2.12 fewer deaths for every 1,000 patients. Of the patients with complications, a 7.47 reduction of patient deaths per 1,000 patients is noted (Kutney-Lee, Sloane, & Aiken, 2013).

Finally, Blegen, Goode, Park, Vaughn, and Spetz published their cross-sectional study of 21 University HealthSystem Consortium hospitals in the *Journal of Nursing Administration*. They note that hospitals with more nurses who have a BSN degree or higher have lower rates of post-op deep vein thrombosis, pressure ulcers, failure to rescue, and congestive heart failure mortality, as well as shorter lengths of stay (Blegen et al., 2013).

Please see the references noted in the back of this book to fully explore these research articles. I encourage you to also explore this topic on your own. There are many more great research articles from various nursing organizations and researchers that further substantiate this point. Go online and search "bachelor's-prepared nurses and patient outcomes" and you will get a plethora of information.

> *"ADN nurses are more clinically prepared when they graduate from school. BSN graduates don't even know the basics."*

Response: While it may take longer to get BSN students up to speed practically at the bedside, they are educated about the entirety of the profession with courses related to informatics, evidence-based practice, and research. This larger knowledge base is proven (see above) to produce better outcomes. Just because a BSN nurse right out of school may never have put in a Foley catheter or has only started a handful of IVs does not mean they are not safe care providers.

> *"ADN nurses can adequately lead the health care team with an associate's degree."*

Response: We all know how it works. The nurse is the care-team coordinator and gatekeeper for the patient. They are running the show from an interdisciplinary standpoint. Everyone from the physician to the chaplain checks with the nurse first. However, did you know that all members of the health care team are required to have a bachelor's degree or higher, except for nurses and respiratory therapists?

Below are the minimum educational requirements for the interdisciplinary team:

- *Physician*: Medical degree (at least eight years of college)
- *Pharmacist*: Doctorate degree (at least six years of college)
- *Physical therapist*: Master's degree (many have doctorate, at least six years of college)
- *Occupational therapist*: Master's degree (some have doctorate, at least six years of college)
- *Speech therapist*: Master's degree (at least six years of college)
- *Nutritionist*: Bachelor's degree (at least four years of college)
- *Case manager*: Bachelor's degree (at least four years of college)
- *Social worker*: Bachelor's degree (at least four years of college)
- *Chaplain*: Bachelor's degree (many masters-. or doctorate-prepared, at least four years of college)
- *Respiratory therapist*: Associate's degree (bachelor's degree available, at least two years of college)

- *Registered nurse*: Associate's degree or bachelor's degree (at least two years of college)

"All BSN programs do is force people to write more papers; it's not practical knowledge that helps our profession."

Response: While BSN programs do require more courses and therefore papers, they provide valuable and essential information related to our profession as a whole. Cramming all of the necessary information for becoming a nurse and passing the NCLEX into two years is a challenge. There simply is not enough time to provide the education that a BSN degree provides. Therefore, ADN programs are forced to focus on getting the nurse ready with the most practical information regarding patient care, not the information that pertains to our profession as a whole (for example, nursing research and informatics courses). Again, it has been proven that these courses and knowledge base mean fewer patient deaths later down the line.

Because of this nationwide initiative, a lot of colleges and universities are stepping up to the plate to provide programs to meet this demand. There are a few options out there for ADN nurses with an RN license.

RN-to-BSN Completion or Bridge Programs

These can be completed completely online, in person, or a combination thereof. Many times you can choose how quickly you would like to complete them (as either a part-time or full-time student). Also, many employers want their nurses to become BSN-prepared, so make sure you check to see what kind of benefits they may offer in regard to tuition reimbursement. Some schools are even partnering with employers to offer discounts as well.

There are also a few schools that have programs where you can take competency exams to get credit for information you already know so you are not taking courses on topics you already have learned on the job. This can shorten the amount of time it takes to obtain the degree and tailor your courses to your needs.

Graduate Degrees and Graduate Preparation in Nursing

There are multiple options and paths for those looking to continue their education past a bachelor's degree. When thinking about graduate school, it is really important to know what you would ultimately like to do. Do you want to be a nurse practitioner? Do you want to work in nursing leadership? Would you like to do research? There are quite a few options out there. Below is a basic explanation of your graduate-level options in the field of nursing. Most of the information below was gathered from "Your Guide to Graduate Nursing Programs," published by the American Association of Colleges of Nursing in 2011.

Master of Science in Nursing (MSN)
There are multiple options for this level, including options for the associate's-prepared nurse. There are many ADN-to-MSN programs available. There is also an option for people who have a bachelor's or graduate degree in a field other than nursing. These can take a little longer, as it takes about two to three years to finish the bachelor's level coursework and to become a licensed nurse in addition to the master's level courses.

There is an option for those who already have a BSN, as well as those who would like to do a dual master's degree and obtain their MSN along with another master's, such as public administration (MPA), health administration (MHA), or even business (MBA).

After obtaining your MSN, you have many options ahead of you. Management, clinical, and collegiate education, as well as involvement in policy and research are all possibilities with an MSN.

Advanced Practice Registered Nurse (APRN)
This graduate level of practice will enable you to work in a clinical setting. While an APRN is not a degree itself, it is a master's-prepared specialty, which requires a license. You can work directly with patients and the medical team to provide care and diagnoses, place orders under your own license, and even perform advanced procedures. There are many different options as an APRN.

> *Nurse practitioners (NPs)*: This degree will enable you to do the aforementioned things in many different settings. You can work within a physician group, a nurse practitioner group, or even have your own independent practice. Many specialties employ NPs, which gives you many options to choose from, similar to bedside nursing.
>
> *Certified registered nurse anesthetists (CRNAs)*: This is a very specific specialization. Entry into these programs is very selective, and the coursework is very rigorous. Most programs will require you to go full-time and will not allow employment outside of the intense

coursework. Also, most programs require applicants to have experience in critical care or the emergency department before entry. Once
completed, you can be an anesthesia provider in any number of cases.
Some work under the supervision of an anesthesiologist and some do
not. This is also currently the highest-paid nursing specialty in our field.

Certified nurse midwives (CNMs): This is another very specific special-
ization within an already specialized patient population. This degree
enables you to provide many services. While CNMs typically focus on
obstetrical and gynecological preventative care, they can also care for
women during childbirth as well as care for the newborn.

Clinical nurse specialist (CNSs): CNSs focus on a specific patient population. From medical–surgical to critical care to behavioral health, these
APRNs are focused on evidence-based practice and have knowledge
related to cost and improvement. According to the AACN's guide,
"The CNS is responsible and accountable for diagnosis and treatment
of health/illness states, disease management, health promotion and
prevention of illness, and risk behaviors among individuals, families,
communities, and groups" (2011, p. 8).

After you attain this level in one of these aforementioned areas, the sky is
the limit! There are so many different and innovative ways to utilize the
degree that I cannot even begin to describe them all here. Just know that
the standard for APRNs is becoming more doctorate-focused. Therefore,
if you're looking into one of these options, you may want to see if there
is a post-master's DNP option available. Education, research, informatics,
administration, public health, forensics, case management, and genetics
are just a few options out there.

Doctorate of Nursing Practice (DNP)

As previously mentioned, the standard for APRNs is shifting from a master's
degree to a doctorate degree. Interestingly enough, the amount of credits
that nurses obtain while working toward their master's degrees is actually
more comparable to a doctorate degree in other health professions. This is
why many nursing programs are moving away from the master's level of
preparedness for various roles and focusing more on the doctorate level.
Some schools no longer offer a master's-level nurse practitioner degree.

This degree would fulfill that new standard. The curriculum is focused
on evidence-based practice, health-systems leadership, and also quality
improvement. Nurses with this degree are great with research and can
take this research and implement its findings at the bedside within a health
system.

The Doctor of Philosophy (PhD) in Nursing

Contrary to popular belief, this degree is not the same as a DNP degree. This degree is more academic and research-focused. Essentially, the PhD-prepared nurse creates the research and thus is more research-oriented and academic, while the DNP-prepared nurse puts this into practice and thus is more practice-oriented. This degree does take longer to complete than the DNP, as there are more credit hours required.

As you can see, there are many options ahead of you as a nurse. This was a basic explanation of options. Please know that there are more available out there, as this list was not exhaustive.

How Do I Know What I Want to Do?

There are a few recommendations that I have for those of you looking to go back to school.

First, decide what exactly you would like to do. Don't put the cart before the horse and just say you want specific letters after your name. Figure out what you would practically like your career to look like first. Once you have decided this, look at the best path to get there. The last thing you want is to go through all the work of getting into college, only to discover it is not what you wanted in the first place, the hours are not sustainable with your life, or you cannot handle the time commitment.

Questions to ask yourself:

1. **What do I want to do every day?** Do you want to interact with patients, nursing students, health care leaders and executives, lawmakers, researchers, or others involved in nursing-related work? Some nurses will be in an office all day doing behind the scenes work, some will travel a lot, some will work directly with patients, some will be in front of a classroom.... You name it.

2. **What kind of hours do I want?** Do you want to work 0800–1700, Monday–Friday, or do you want shift work? Is being on-call something you are okay with?

3. **Are my goals not only obtainable, but also sustainable?** After all the work has been done and you start your new role with your new degree, would this be a job you will want to do for years to come? Are the hours, the type of work, the patients, the location, and so on, all things that you can handle? Factoring in all of your life commitments, how will this fit into your life? Will this satisfy your personal and professional needs?

4. **Can my family and I handle this financially?** I know many programs have loans, grants, and scholarships; however, you must have a clear

financial picture and plan in front of you before making this decision. While it is easy to take out a loan, it is a very long road in postgraduation repayment. Calculate your possible monthly loan payment, along with a low estimate of your new monthly salary. Does this fit? Can you make this work? School can be stressful, as can starting a new job with a new role. Adding on an insurmountable financial burden, which could have been avoided with the appropriate research and planning, can make that stress unbearable. Do your financial research. Do not make the mistake of getting a set of credentials behind your name from a specific school if it will leave you and your family in financial stress for years to come. There are many affordable options out there.

5. **Can I make the time commitment to this potential degree?** Going back to school full-time and working full-time is very challenging, especially when you have other personal responsibilities, like caring for children or your parents. When talking to potential schools, really understand what the time commitment of part-time versus full-time will look like and practically apply that to your life today. You want to approach this in a way where you are taking on manageable chunks and not living in this constant state of being stressed and overwhelmed. Keep in mind that this may mean delaying getting the degree by taking it slower. Maybe you want to get an MSN but need to go part-time. This may mean it can take as long as four years to complete the degree. Therefore, plan four years ahead. Can you continue this time and financial commitment for four years? Will there be periods of time you may be able to take an additional course or two? Do you have anything coming up (for example, potentially starting a family) that may delay completion? These things are important to consider. They should not deter you from your degree, but it is important to practically consider all aspects of your life and commitments for the potential duration of the academic course to make the best decision possible.

6. **Will I be okay with the potential salary?** Some degrees and positions offer very high salaries while others are not in the same ballpark. It is important to consider if the money you invest into the degree will be worth it to you based on your earning potential after obtaining the degree. Again, it is crucial to factor in potential monthly loan payments (and all other monthly expenses) with your new prospective salary.

You should exhaust all of these questions when looking at a degree. Many schools would love you to be their next student. However, only you know the answers to these questions. Only you really know your needs and goals and how to practically address them. These schools do not. Please keep that in mind when working with advisors.

It is also important to thoroughly discuss this with any loved ones that may be walking through this journey with you. Your spouse, your parents, important support people, or even your children are essential people to bring into the conversation. Trying to get a degree without any emotional, spiritual, or practical support can be a recipe for an overworked, overwhelmed, and underappreciated nurse. Make sure you are vocalizing your goals, the support you need to obtain them, and how this will fit into your family dynamic.

School Shopping

There are so many things to consider when picking a school. Think of it like a long-term relationship, because you will be dealing with them for years to come. Remember: *you* are the student and this is your degree. You have the power and right to ask as many questions as possible from all potential schools. Do not feel like you are bugging advisors with your questions—they must be answered. You must fully understand what you are getting yourself into and what to expect.

The Biggest Mistake You Can Make

Please do not have a general idea of what you would like to do, apply to a few schools, and go with the first one that sends you an acceptance letter. While it feels great to see that you were accepted into a school, it does not necessarily mean it will be the best overall fit for you. Make sure you are doing the appropriate planning and research before diving headfirst into the depths of education. I highly recommend creating a chart comparing all of your potential schools.

Requirements for Acceptance

Some schools require much more than others to be accepted. It is important to know for those of you looking at getting your BSN if you will need to retake any prerequisite courses. Some schools do not require this, while others do. Some require various science and math courses to have been completed in the last five years. This may mean retaking courses, which will add to your timeline and budget. Please make sure to figure prerequisite courses, if they are needed, into your planning.

Furthermore, some advanced degrees have specific requirements regarding your nursing experience. Research the websites of each potential school for any clinical or practical experience they require. Also, it is important to know the minimum acceptable GPA as well as whether the GRE is required. Some nursing schools do not require the GRE. However, if your school does, you must add that into your timeline and expenses as well. You will need to pay for study materials as well as for the exam itself and make a time commitment to study.

Finances

Understand exactly how much your degree will cost. Figure in all scholarships (there are many available for nurses), grants, and loans. Many employers offer tuition reimbursement, and some work with specific schools to offer additional discounts. There are also a lot of options out there for military personnel, so make sure you understand all benefits granted to you so that you can fully maximize them.

It is important to know not only your final cost for tuition but also the cost for books and additional fees. These can really add up! Many schools are pretty competitive with their prices, but this does not mean all of them are about the same.

Quality of the School

Is it accredited? When is its accreditation up for renewal? Is it in the process of renewal at this time, and if so, how is it going? Where does it rank nationally? If you are looking at a specific graduate degree, is the faculty in line with your goals? Look online at the faculty, get their contact information, and reach out. Ask specific questions to get a feel for them and their passion within the field of nursing.

Logistics of the Program

Are you someone who needs to physically be in the classroom, or are you an online student through and through? Obviously if you are looking at being in a program in which you need to attend classes, location will be a major factor in this decision. Many programs are online, and some offer the option to be half online and half in the classroom. Decide what will work best for your learning needs.

If you go with an online program, make sure you are paying attention to the website, application process, and online services. If you are going to be fully online, you want to make sure that the program has a website and online services that you can easily navigate and participate in. Check and see what the technical requirements are and if you have the appropriate equipment at home. If you do not, make sure you add purchasing that equipment (computer, webcam, printer, and so forth) into your budget.

One thing I like to make sure is clear is how I will access their online journals and databases. Many of these degrees require utilization of many sources for various posts, papers and other assignments. How will this school enable your access to these? Is it part of the actual school's library or website, or will you have to go out of your online learning modules and programs to another one to access this information?

As you can tell, going back to continue your education can be an extremely worthwhile and rewarding process. However, it is essential to complete the research beforehand to make sure you are going after the best degree at the best school for you. Many people have very different financial situations, aspirations, and commitments at home. Just because one school and degree was perfect for one person does not mean it will work out the same for another.

6

Extending Your Professional Credentials: Organizations, Certifications, and Conferences

Another way to dig deeper into the profession of nursing is to become involved in professional organizations. Through these organizations, one can become a nationally certified nurse, attend national conferences, and have access to many continuing education opportunities, chapter meetings, and publications.

National Professional Nursing Organizations: What They Are, Why They're Important

Most nursing specialties have a professional organization associated with them in addition to some of the nationwide professional organizations for nurses. For example, I am a neuroscience critical care nurse. Therefore, I am a member of the American Association of Critical Care Nurses (AACN), the American Association of Neuroscience Nurses (AANN), and the American Nurses Association (ANA). Every single month I get professional nursing journals from each of these organizations that talk about some of the latest evidenced-based practice occurring in my field, some issues or challenges facing the profession, and recommended reading and other interesting articles. I am able to attend chapter meetings, if I so choose, as well as explore the many online resources all of these organizations provide.

Staying involved with your respective nursing organizations allows you, as a bedside nurse, to have your finger on the pulse of your specialty on a national level. You can read about a research study occurring halfway across the country that may benefit your patient population and potentially implement these findings on your unit. Being aware of the latest research, best practices, and trends across the country consistently educates and enables you to profoundly impact patient care and outcomes—you just have to use this knowledge. Having regular and easy access to the latest research empowers you, the bedside nurse, to effect policy change. You can utilize this information in so many ways, from educating other nurses in staff meetings, to creating your own research projects, to bringing your ideas to best-practice teams within your organizations to actually change policies to reflect the latest research. The power nurses have through these organizations is amazing.

This does not just apply to the unit level, however. This applies to the national level as well. Many professional nursing organizations are involved with health policy legislation. The American Nurses Association, American Association of the Colleges of Nurses, and the Nursing Organizations Alliance are just a few organizations that are heavily involved in legislation. You do not have to be a nurse with decades of experience and multiple credentials behind your name to get involved and make a difference.

The best place to find out what organization(s) would best fit you and your practice would probably be the Nursing Organizations Alliance. They have a comprehensive list of all professional nursing organizations with a link to each of their sites.

Membership benefits can vary from organization to organization, but they generally include a monthly publication of some sort, access to their online resources and newsletters, and also invitations to chapter meetings. Depending on your location, there are many local chapters of professional organizations.

Most professional organizations do require members to pay annual dues. These allow the organization to continue functioning. Again, these vary from organization to organization. However, many health care facilities want their nurses to be involved and will reimburse dues for professional organizations! I personally have not had to pay for dues out of my own pocket yet, as they have all been reimbursed because my employer provides this benefit.

I am a big proponent of these organizations. They give you a bigger picture of nursing outside of your unit. When you work in the same environment day in and day out, it is hard not to develop tunnel vision and get focused on the tasks at hand. However, there is so much more to the profession. Research, legislation, and policy all drive nursing practice, and if you want to have a say in how and why you do what you do with your patients every shift, you must step back from the bedside and see what is going on in the rest of the profession. These organizations are a great place to start because it can be overwhelming when you start looking around online. You are able start with what directly impacts the patients that you know the most about and then go from there.

National Certifications and the Organizations That Award Them

Many certification and professional organizations offer certifications for nurses. Generally speaking, most nursing fields and specialties have a certification that is applicable to them. Basically this means that if you meet the requirements to sit for the exam (typically a certain amount of years of experience within that specialty), then you may do so. Passing this very difficult and rigorous certification exam signifies that you are a nationally certified nurse in your specialty. This indicates that you have a certain level of expertise within your specialty and are dedicated to being educated and knowledgeable about what affects your patient population.

Additionally, this will add credentials to your name. For example, being a neurosciences critical care nurse, there are multiple certifications that I am eligible to take. I first decided to take my critical care certification exam, which was very difficult. My credentials became Kati Kleber, BSN RN CCRN. In addition, there are two more certifications for which I am eligible. I can take the SCRN (stroke certified registered nurse) and the CNRN (certified neuroscience registered nurse). If I were to take and pass all three exams, my credentials would be Kati Kleber, BSN RN CCRN SCRN CNRN. Phew! What an educated mouthful!

Therefore, depending on where you currently work and your experience level in that area, you may be able to sit for a certification exam, if not multiple. This is a prestigious achievement in nursing and highly celebrated. It is so highly celebrated that there is even a national Certified

Nurses Day, which is March 19th of every year. Some health care facilities even provide bonuses to certified nurses. Many reimburse for the certification exam as well.

National Conferences

In addition to certifications, publications, involvement in legislation, and research, many national nursing organizations hold a national conference. I confess: I am a bit of a conference geek. In my mere five years as a registered nurse, I have been to six different conferences. I love them; I believe they are so valuable. My favorite conferences have been the National Teaching Institute and Critical Care Exposition (NTI) conferences, which the American Association of Critical Care Nurses hosts every year. There were over 8,000 critical care nurses in one conference center when I went in 2015 to San Diego, California. They had large sessions with everyone in attendance with amazing keynote speakers. Like many conferences, they had breakout sessions as well. You are able take a look at the scheduled ahead of time and figure out which sessions you would like to go to. Going to these sessions provides you with real, practical knowledge that you can bring back to your unit and apply. They also provide you with continuing education hours, so you can get many that are necessary to maintain your nursing license in just a few days.

Conferences are invigorating, renewing, and enlightening. They really help you feel and understand the importance of your role as a nurse and what you can do to become better. I felt very valued and empowered to make a difference for my patients and myself after attending every single one of those conferences. They can be expensive to attend, but many hospitals will reimburse or cover some expenses if you plan in advance. If you have never been to one, I highly recommend going, even it means paying for some of it yourself. With early planning, some financial support from your facility, and making sure you get some good deals on food and travel, they are well worth the money.

I encourage you to check out the professional nursing organizations that are applicable to your practice. Regardless of your field, the American Nurses Association and your respective state's organization, through which you also have membership to ANA (mine is the North Carolina Nurses Association), are great places to start. Go to the ANA website (http://www.nursingworld.org), go to the upper-right corner, and click on About ANA, Find Your State, and FAQs to become acquainted.

I also encourage you to ask other nurses on your unit if they or anyone else there is in a professional organization, which one (or two), and if they are, consider asking for help by walking you through the process of becoming involved.

7

Moving into the Extraordinary: Magnet Designation and Shared Governance

When I was going through my nursing residency program right out of school, I was told about something called "Magnet" and shared governance at my hospital. I was pretty overwhelmed with all of the new things I was learning, so it was definitely something I put on the backburner at the time. They told me that Magnet was a prestigious nursing designation that only 6% of hospitals in the country had; however, I did not fully understand what that meant.

Once I was off orientation and starting to really grasp the picture of what it meant to be a nurse on my unit, my manager asked me to be our unit representative on various committees. When I started in nursing, I had no idea how many committees for nursing there really are. There are so many. Best practice committees, shared governance committees, Magnet Champion committees, preceptor groups—the list goes on and on. I can't remember why, but I just thought that once you were a nurse on a unit, that was it. You came in and took care of your patients, and that was that; there was no behind-the-scenes action that fueled what I do at the bedside. I just figured there was some big group of people in an office somewhere who dictated what nurses are supposed to do, and we just did what we were told and did not have a say in it. Oh, how wrong I was!

There is much more to being a nurse than that. I started to realize that the policies and procedures that I had been looking up all through orientation were developed and edited by nurses. The recommendations to changes in our electronic charting systems were gathered and presented by nurses. It was nurses who completed all the development and implementation of our clinical ladder program and nurse residency program. Nurses were doing research at the bedside to make policy recommendations and changes. I just always assumed that these changes all came from the top down, and we came into work, followed the rules, and left. I started to realize that we have a big part in the majority of decisions that dictate how we do our job. We sit at the table, and in many cases, we are the entire table.

When I started to put these pieces together, I got excited. I started to get involved in the various committees, and my understanding of nursing quickly deepened. One of the first issues my manager asked me to get involved in was in being our unit's Magnet Champion. Through this, I quickly learned what a big deal Magnet designation really is. I discuss it briefly over the next few pages, then turn to the idea of shared governance in nursing, which is closely linked with, but not dependent on, Magnet.

Magnet Designation

So: what is "Magnet designation"? "The ANCC Magnet Recognition Program® is viewed around the world as the ultimate seal of quality and confidence. Magnet organizations are recognized for superior nursing processes and quality patient care, which lead to the highest levels of safety, quality, and patient satisfaction" (ANCC, 2016b). At first, that was just a boilerplate sentence to me. I did not really understand what that meant. However, since I first became a nurse in 2010, I have had the privilege of working at two Magnet hospitals. I have seen the immense amount of work and time that goes into obtaining this designation first hand.

This designation is more than paperwork and meetings. It involves the entire organization, not just the nurses at the bedside. It takes years to go on the "Magnet journey," more formally known as "The Journey to Magnet Excellence."

The Magnet journey consists of three steps. (For more details on each step, go to http://www.nursecredentialing.org/MagnetJourney.) The first is to analyze your gaps. The organization looks at its current data and performance and develops action plans to improve. This can include things like increasing the number of bachelor's-prepared and certified nurses at your facility, establishing shared governance, or increasing your RN satisfaction rate. Honestly, when I first started, I had no idea that people were not only looking at this data but also caring about it.

Next, you must gain assistance from the assigned Senior Program Analyst, a representative from the Magnet staff who assists throughout the process with clarifying questions about documentation and requirements. Gaining assistance will continue throughout the process.

The final and most intense step is to transform the culture. Staff must be educated; infrastructure must be developed to support the recommended programs (such as shared governance, peer review, nursing research, evidence-based practice); the staff must become engaged in professional development; a timeline must be developed; achievements must be recognized and evaluated; the organization of the culture must be inspected as it evolves and addressed appropriately. Top leadership at the organization must be closely involved in this process.

This process is so in-depth, thorough, and important that many facilities actually employ someone to spearhead this as their entire job.

So, why should you, your unit, and your hospital care? Why should pretty much an entire staff do all of this work to get this designation? The bottom line is patient safety. Magnet-designated hospitals have better outcomes. Period. Per the ANCC website, "studies assessing links between the work environment for nurses and the patient safety climate find Magnet hospital experience increased patient satisfaction, decreased mortality rates, decreased pressure ulcers, decreased falls, and improved quality" (ANCC, 2016a). Please see the special reference list on page 92 for some sources that substantiate this point.

Becoming a Magnet-designated hospital is not easy. It takes a lot of work from the entire organization, not just one person or the top-level executives. The boots-on-the-ground nurses must be involved. One of the best ways for any nurse to be actively involved in this process is to sit on one of the previously mentioned committees and councils. I have been involved in various groups, but the one that I have found that had the most impact on my day-to-day work has been shared governance.

Shared Governance in Nursing

This can look different at different facilities, but the concept is the same throughout. Now, I know what you may be thinking: "I don't want to get involved in anything else at work; I am too busy." However, I cannot overemphasize the value of shared governance. It is worth talking to your manager to see if schedule adjustments can be made so that you are not overwhelmed with your regular work schedule in addition to going to these meetings. It is so enlightening, empowering, and refreshing.

In his article, "From Bedside to Boardroom" in the *Online Journal of Issues in Nursing,* Robert Hess (2004) defines shared governance as "an organizational model through which nurses control their practice as well as influence administrative areas." The actual structure of shared governance at each health care facility can vary widely, but this is the basic definition and function.

Why is this important? Why should facilities spend time, money, and effort to get a shared governance model up and running at a health care facility? A study of over 3,500 nurses dating all the way to 1988 concluded that autonomy over nursing judgment is an essential aspect of nursing practice. (Huey & Hartley, p. 181–188).

Think about this in how it relates to policy and procedure development. You, as a bedside nurse, use these policies and procedures to guide your patient care every single shift. You are the one using them day in and day out; you know what works and what does not, and what questions arise while utilizing them. While there are people behind the scenes, who are frequently also nurses, creating these policies and ensuring they are appropriately structured from a legal standpoint, there must be people involved in their development who actually utilize them. Shared governance bridges that gap. It is up to you, the bedside nurse, to have a say in your practice, to give input where it is desperately needed, and to influence how you give care.

The basic purpose of shared governance, no matter the structure, is to "gather managers and staff together to make decisions" (Hess, 2004). Put another way: "Shared governance is collaboration, whether in scheduling staff, educating new staff, or implementing evidence-based practice. It involves teamwork, problem-solving, and accountability, with the goals of improved staff satisfaction, productivity, and patient outcomes. It is working together to make decisions that affect nursing practice and patient care. It is working with other disciplines for the good of the patient. It is collaborating to improve nursing practice" (Bonsall, 2011). Multiple models and structures are available, and I will not outline all of them here. There are many wonderful books and resources available that can outline the specifics and provide practical information about starting and maintaining shared governance at your facility. Please see the recommended reading list at the back of this book to get started.

What kind of changes can shared governance make? It is important to understand that change on an organizational scale does not just happen overnight, from one suggestion from one employee. To change practice, research must be utilized to substantiate the change as well as prove that it is financially responsible. For example, if you are noticing that your central line–associated blood stream infections (CLABSIs) are quickly going up, you may sit down with your shared governance group to see how you can address this problem. Maybe someone in the group suggests purchasing new technology to enable nurses to start IVs easier and therefore decrease the number of central lines.

Theoretically this sounds good, but you will not get an administrative team to invest a large sum of money on a facility-wide scale if they are not certain it will be worth the money. Therefore, you and your team pull a literature review together about the product you're interested in. After figuring in the cost of the equipment and the training required to utilize it properly and maintain this skill, you and your team note that the potential benefits do not outweigh the time, effort, and cost. However, through your research you note that hospitals with vascular access teams report significantly lower CLASBI rates than hospitals without them. You procure more research to further substantiate this through another literature review.

After you have compiled research and potential cost savings, you and your team of bedside nurse coworkers bring this information to the administrative team and say, "The problem of increasing CLASBI rates was brought to us, and after looking at different options to address this, we discovered that the research substantiates investment in the development of a vascular access team. We currently lose _____ amount of dollars on these infections annually because our current rate is _____. However, hospitals with vascular access teams report an average infection rate of _____. If we dropped our rate from our average to their average, we stand to save approximately _____. A rough estimate of the cost of this team is _____. Our committee would be interested in piloting this program on a few units and creating a research study for publication. If our research further substantiates the existing research, we believe investing in the creation of a vascular access team would be beneficial for the nurse, the patient, and the organization."

Wow. You have just impressed your executive team! A problem was identified and not only did you come up a solution, you were able to back it up with existing research, suggest creating additional research, and also present the benefits of the solution in terms of dollars. This is how change happens.

If you are thinking about getting involved in an existing council, I highly encourage it. I am sure there are many procedures or policies in your unit or area that you think could be better or more efficient. Your voice matters, your role matters, and you have the power to influence change.

If you want to get shared governance started at your facility, please make sure to read and research the best way to go about this. Different organizations have different needs, and what works at a friend's hospital down the street might not work functionally at yours. Establishing a shared governance council is definitely a marathon, not a sprint. It requires structure and administrative support, and the staff has to really buy in and see it as an added value to them and their patients.

To bring this around full circle with Magnet, I want to reiterate that shared governance is an aspect of obtaining and maintaining the Magnet designation. When the ANCC Magnet team is evaluating a hospital for this designation, they look for shared governance to be established and active as part of the structural empowerment aspect of the Magnet Model. The other four parts of the Model are transformational leadership, exemplary professional practice, empirical outcomes, and new knowledge, innovations, and improvements (ANCC, 2016c). Magnet and shared governance go hand in hand.

8

Dealing with Negative Coworkers: Steps to a Positive Unit Culture

This entire book has been about furthering your career, jumping into professional development in nursing, and enhancing your work life. However, as with anything in life, when people are trying to make things better for themselves, others may not have great things to say. This always perplexes me, but it does occur in many professions when people try to better themselves personally. Therefore, it is not about avoiding these people and interactions, but about dealing with them when they occur.

We all know what negative coworkers are like. We all know how they severely impact the culture on the nursing unit. You dread seeing their name on the schedule the same day as yours. You hate to tell them they're floating today because you know you'll get an earful when you're just trying to do your job. You hate to tell them they're getting the next patient, even though it is their turn, because you know they will complain. Every time change occurs, they complain constantly and do not offer solutions.

They commiserate with others who live their lives in the same way. It's terrible when more than one of them are working the same shift as you because they spend more time complaining and commiserating than actually taking care of patients. They hang out at the nurse's station with their irritable attitudes, while others are answering their alarms and call bells. Because of their commanding presence, you do not feel comfortable confronting them or holding them accountable. You wait and pray for management to step in.

Nursing units function like teams: We rely heavily on each other when things get busy or chaotic. We should not sit in our little silos, do our work on only our patients, and go home. It just does not work like that. We must work together to meet the demands on the unit every day. It is simply absurd for one person to think they can take care of their entire patient load by themselves. I believe this is why people are hesitant to confront others when they display destructive behavior. When it has been seven hours since you've sat down or gone to the bathroom and you know Negative Nancy is all caught up, you want to be able to ask her to do a few things for you so you can get caught up too. But if you're on her bad side, not only is she not going to help but she will talk negatively about you to others as well. It is all about survival in a negative culture. People shy away from holding negative people accountable because of the repercussions and lack of change. It just ends up not being worth it.

The worst part of this is that they are engraining this negativity into the culture of your unit. Surprisingly, these overly negative people are often among the informal leaders on the unit. They are good technical nurses, know how to care for patients, and have a commanding presence. Therefore, when new nurses join the team, they quickly learn that, in order to fit in with the culture and the experienced people on the floor, they have to be negative. People who are not very negative people are suddenly negative just to fit in and assimilate into the culture of this unit. This is a dangerous spiral.

In this culture of negativity, change—when it inevitably occurs—is always met with resistance. This is especially frustrating when the change was well-communicated and supported by research. You feel like no one can win. Most people spend their shift accommodating attitudes instead of taking good care of patients.

Does this sound familiar? Sorry if I gave you hypertension from just reading the description. It is important to know that this is not how nursing units should function, even if "it's always been that way." This is not conducive to safe patient care and nursing satisfaction.

Nursing units should encourage professional development, not just from the top down, but laterally as well. Nurses should be encouraging each other get involved, learn more, adapt well, and just do the best they can for their patients every day. Nurses going above and beyond should not be met with resistance, but with excitement and encouragement. Therefore, if you find yourself meeting some resistance, here are some helpful hints to dealing with it.

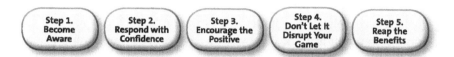

Step 1. Become Aware

It is important to realize the cultural climate of your unit. If you are so deeply immersed in it that you cannot clearly see if it is negative, positive, or just apathetic, it is hard to address the need, or even know there is one. Try to step back and see how people interact. Think about how you feel about work. Do you enjoy going in? Do you look on the schedule to see with whom you're working because there are about four to five people you just hate to be scheduled with? Do you find yourself picking up the slack of others but not feeling comfortable confronting them about it because "it's just not worth it"? Have you just learned to deal with it and care less?

If you are going to go against the grain and do something a little different, it helps to be aware of the climate. If you are aware of the culture, you will be less likely to take what they say personally. When people cut down others for no good reason, it is typically out of their own hurt and insecurities. Being aware of that allows you to remove yourself a bit from the situation and have a better understanding of why they may be acting that way. This awareness can also just help you survive in a negative culture. Allow yourself to step outside of the situations and relationships and think about why people respond the way they do. It helps you not to take it personally, and therefore, it will not affect you as much. You are able to respond with more grace, kindness, and wisdom rather than snapping back and making the culture worse. You move on faster and can focus on what does matter: your patient care, teamwork, and your professional development.

Step 2. Respond with Confidence

Confidence is key in the midst of negativity. Combine that with your newfound understanding of the unit culture, and you are good to go! There will probably be nurses on your unit who have been there for 15 years who have never been to a meeting, read research studies, sat on a committee, or done more than the minimum. Someone jumping on the professional development train might seem odd or unnecessary to them, or it may bring out some insecurity because they are not doing the same. Do not let someone else's negativity or insecurities keep you from achieving your goals. It is completely fine if they do not want to participate; you have no control over their actions. What you do have control over is your actions and how you respond to theirs.

These situations can get awkward. You are all hanging out at the nurse's station, and someone makes a backhanded comment, starts asking why you do all that extra work, or says that nothing ever gets accomplished anyway so there's no need to waste time. It is in front of a bunch of others so you feel like you need to say something good. I think it is important to keep these interactions short and sweet and always make sure you are taking the high road. A simple response like, "I just don't think people can complain unless they are going to be part of the solution, which is why I go to these meetings," can go a long way. It does not degrade the person, even though that is what they are trying to do to you, but communicates that you have accountability and are not going to join their negative party.

Regardless of how negative someone can be, I personally have made a commitment to myself to be unapologetically positive. If someone wants to live their life being negative, seeing all of the problems and complaining about them, while refusing to adjust to change and therefore making everyone else's life miserable, that is their choice. But it will never be mine.

I choose to walk into work with a good attitude. While some days are easier than others, I choose to see the positive side of things. I also know how to communicate concerns in a respectful way, not in a way that brings others down. It is important to hold on to this when people question you or are consistently negative. They may be a smart and experienced nurse, but if they walk into work every day with a cloud over their head and a mission to make everyone else miserable as well, refuse to take part in that. Be conscious of it and be able to identify it so you are able to see the situation for what it is and separate yourself.

Step 3. Encourage the Positive

When the negative people are actually being positive and constructive, engage with them. Talk more about it, be more interested, and place value on it. When they begin being negative, step away if you do not feel comfortable calling it out directly. Become less engaged, do not wallow with them and create joy from their misery. Soon, they will learn that their old way of complaining, cutting down, and being negative is not the way to get attention on the unit. Positivity will be what gets them an audience; negativity will cause people to disperse.

When they start to talk negatively about a coworker, bring up a positive thing for every negative thing they say.

"I can't believe they didn't even know how to change a central line dressing! I mean, how long have they been a nurse!?" they say, hoping for someone else to chime in with something else they've noticed.

"She's new to critical care. It may take her a few times to remember how to do it. Have you seen her start an IV though? She slammed an 18 gauge in on this dialysis patient that all of us tried to stick and none of us could get," is a potential response.

Another option of something to say within that situation is to call it out in a subtle type of way. When a negative comment is brought up, saying something like, "Man, I hope no one talks about me like that when I screw up!" can put things into perspective.

Again, confidence is key. Refuse to participate. Be bigger than the negative culture and people. Be aware and refuse to reward it.

Step 4. Don't Let It Disrupt Your Game

When people are not thrilled with your participation or maybe don't fully understand it, do not let it interrupt what you've got going on. Continue to work with confidence on the things that you have decided are important to you and add value to your life and career.

Take those times when people question your reasoning for furthering your career and turn them into teachable moments. Utilize these situations to enlighten people, not to force or shame them into doing more for their professional development. I find it very valuable when I see others explain the benefits of what they are doing without shoving it down someone else's throat. Presenting something in a way that says, "I've been on this committee for about six months and really enjoy it because they take my opinion seriously with policy change. A policy was recently changed because of my input, and I think that's pretty awesome," can go a lot farther than "You need to just come to the meeting. It will be good for you. I just love it so much!"

Also keep in mind that your enthusiasm and general increased interest, whether you say something directly to someone or not, speaks volumes. Engaging in meetings, talking about them, getting your certification, and speaking with nursing leadership about change can inspire people without you even trying. Maybe there are a few nurses on your unit who have thought about getting their certification for years but viewed it as this unobtainable dream or aspiration. Once they see you from afar studying for the test, passing, and getting to put those letters behind your name, they will realize that it is not an unrealistic goal. It inspires others. It encourages them. It is especially inspiring when you do it with confidence.

I have heard the occasional response, "Why are you wasting your time with a certification? It's not like we get paid more." I personally value certification and respect others that achieve this goal, regardless of the compensation behind it. Therefore, when people come at me in not the kindest way, I do not take it personally. We clearly prioritize our professional values differently, and that's okay; I do not want to waste my time being offended when they do not see the value in something that I do.

Step 5. Reap the Benefits

It's really interesting to see how immersing yourself in continued personal improvement spills over into your patient care. When things change or new and challenging problems arise, you no longer view them as this massive stress-inducing situation. They suddenly become something that you can handle or troubleshoot with confidence and ease. As you get more involved in the interworkings of your facility, you learn the resources inside and out. You know whom to call with various situations. Also, when you, as an end user/bedside nurse, see things that need to be changed, you know what to do in that situation as well. Much less time is spent spinning your nursing wheels. You can identify a problem and a solution and bring it to the appropriate authority promptly instead of complaining about it for months hoping management finally listens.

I also make it a point not to feel like it is solely my responsibility to change the mind of someone who is not a fan of what I'm doing. That can really hang people up when they feel like it is their duty to convince others what

When Negativity Goes Toxic: Incivility and Bullying in the Workplace and What You Can Do About It

You might be surprised to learn that many of the impolite, disrespectful, and disruptive behaviors and actions that I have described in this chapter can be considered as something other than simply negative. They are viewed by an increasing number of nurses as one part of—think of it as unpleasant and unconstructive leading edge into—a spectrum of inappropriate workplace behavior and actions. One that can start with incivility, then segue into (or at least encourage) harassment, and even bullying. If this sounds extreme and alarmist... here is how the American Nurses Association brings it together (the italics are mine):

> Incivility and bullying in nursing is prevalent in all settings. *Incivility* is one or more *rude, discourteous*, or *disrespectful* actions that may or may not have a negative intent behind them. *Bullying*, which ANA defines as 'repeated, unwanted harmful actions intended to *humiliate, offend* and *cause distress* in the recipient,' is a very serious issue that threatens patient safety, RN safety, and the nursing professional as a whole. (ANA, 2016)

That is from a part of ANA's website on workplace health and safety that focuses to workplace incivility, bullying, and violence ... and where a variety of resources are available. One is ANA's position statement on this topic, where you'll learn that one basis for this is our own profession's code of ethics.

ANA's *Code of Ethics for Nurses with Interpretive Statements* states that nurses are required to "create an ethical environment and culture of civility and kindness, treating colleagues, co-workers, employees, students, and others with dignity and respect" (ANA, 2015, p. 4). Much as we would our patients.

Civil behavior, mutual respect and trust, kindness, thoughtfulness for others are at the core of any healthy and sustaining relationship. Why would we be any different with our coworkers?

they are doing is worth the time and effort. While it is great to communicate to others the value of your decisions, it is not your duty to drag others down this road kicking and screaming. People will be able to tell just from your genuine interest, your calm and respectful attitude, and the benefits you reap from your decisions exactly how valuable professional development is. They will see something in you that they want for themselves. And they will begin to ask about it. Some may not ask in the nicest way, but nonetheless, they will still inquire because it is different to them. People will start to think, "I've been here for 10 years and never enjoyed my job as much as this nurse who has been here for a mere 2 years. What are they doing that's so different? I'm more experienced, have more friends on the unit, and the doctors all know me by name. What gives?"

That may lead to them actually asking you about the things you have decided to become involved in. Now, keep in mind, they may not ask in the most polite way. In these situations, remember why you wanted to get started on this professional development journey and confidently hold on to that. When someone comes at you negatively and seemingly devalues something that is really important to you and that you've worked really hard on, it can be challenging not to be offended. Try to view these opportunities as teaching moments, moments to leave a little mustard seed of inspiration and encouragement. Rarely will you convince someone to dive headfirst into professional development with one conversation, but you can slowly start to inspire them. This inspiration will come not only from the words you say but the respectful and encouraging way in which you say them, your refusal to jump on the negativity bandwagon, and the genuine interest you are exhibiting to this negative person.

9

From One Nurse to Another: My Challenge to You

Throughout my growth as a nurse, I have met many people that view our profession in this "us versus them" manner. It's the nurses versus the patients, nurses versus the medical team, nurses versus management, or even the nurses versus the nurses on another unit. This must stop. We are all one team with one person at the center: the patient. While we are trained as advocates, that should not delineate us from the other essential members of the health care team and the massive amount of people supporting them. We must learn to work together, not fight against one another.

Becoming more deeply involved in professional development will slowly remove that "I always know what's best and I have to fight everyone from other disciplines to get what I need for my patients" attitude. Once that is gone, it is so liberating. You start to value the roles of others more as you deepen your understanding of the interworkings of the hospital. That constant level of distrust dissipates. You are still able to communicate with discernment and advocate appropriately when it is necessary, but you do not approach others like they are out to do the easiest thing, move along, and not really care. And when you do come across people who act like that, you are able to gracefully educate them and advocate, rather than be angry about it for days and further strengthen your wall of distrust.

I encourage you to think of delivering patient care as a collaborative process in which a large team of people are working together for your patients instead of you fighting all of them. It is wonderful and encouraging to truly recognize this and see health care differently. You have a much deeper appreciation for every discipline and the expertise each brings to the table. It honestly makes your job much easier to rely on these people to support and enhance the patient's experience.

Therefore, I challenge you to try something new. I challenge you to just take that first step toward a goal you have been thinking about but just are not sure how to do it or if you even want to. Ask others who are involved about how to practically go about this at your hospital. And if people are not engaged or involved, pave a new way! Just because your unit is disengaged does not mean you must be. Sit down with your manager and tell them your goals. I encourage you to get on social media and see firsthand some of the amazing things nurses are doing all over the world because they decided it was important to them. They did not wait for someone else on their unit to do it—they just jumped in to what they saw as valuable.

Make It the Career You Always Dreamed Of

You have the power to make your nursing career exactly what you want it to be. Gone are the days when you just went to nursing school to become a bedside nurse, kept your head down, and went to work every day. There is so much more to nursing than that. You just have to jump out there and see what gives you personal and professional job satisfaction, what makes you enjoy clocking into work, and what makes you look forward to being there. Maybe you like caring for your patient population, but you are getting complacent. Take some time and think about what would be interesting to you, what you would enjoy. Sit down with your manager, someone within your organization, or someone in nursing that you really look up to and talk it out. Figure out the best way to go about achieving your goals.

I firmly believe that life and work are not meant to just be "getting through." Every single day should add value to your life, even if it is mundane. There should be purpose behind your life and your decisions. If work is becoming something that you dread or you are counting down the hours until you get to go home, you are missing a big part of your life.

I challenge you to figure out what changes in your career you need to make to turn going to work something you genuinely enjoy—something you enjoy so much that it does not seem like work, where you're not counting down the hours until you go home.

No one will do this for you. It is not up to your employer, your school, your family, or your friends. It is up to you to make your career what you want it to be. All of those people out there who enjoy their jobs and their lives are living with intention. They are discovering what gives them joy and going after it. They are not waiting for things to hopefully unfold or for situations to present themselves. They are boldly going after their heart's desires. They are unapologetically confident about what they want. They are facing obstacles with grit and determination.

There is this common misconception that the difference between these people and the rest of the world is circumstance. But life is not about waiting for the right circumstances to present themselves, and then BOOM, life is good and fulfilling. It is about *creating* these circumstances. People hear stories of how someone was "discovered" or just fell into this amazing job and life. Those situations are so rare; they are the exception and not the rule. It is not how life works. Creating these circumstances takes work. It takes failure. It takes putting yourself out there. And most importantly, it takes knowing what you want and unapologetically and fiercely going for it. So, if you are just waiting around for things to happen for you—stop! You are wasting precious time.

While some people may come across more challenges than others, what sets those successful people apart is their determination, accountability, and resiliency. Chances are, there are people out there who have it much worse than you, and there are also many others who have had fewer obstacles. Either way, this should never deter you from your dreams.

Life is not about comparing ourselves to one another to see who had the easiest path, using that to justify why they have achieved their goals, and wallowing that we have not had the same experience. The time you spend comparing yourself to others is time wasted. The time you spend waiting for something to happen to you like it happened to someone you know is time wasted. The time you spend feeling bad about your current circumstances is time wasted.

So, nurse colleague of mine, I challenge you. I challenge you to create the circumstances that would make your career what you always dreamed it to be. Only you have the power to do this. With your nursing license and your determination, nothing can stop you.

Be bold, be confident, and be unapologetic about the nurse you want to become. It is up to you to take that first courageous and daring step.

References

American Association of Colleges of Nursing. (2011). *Your guide to graduate nursing programs.* Retrieved from http://www.aacn.nche.edu/publications/brochures/GradStudentsBrochure.pdf

American Nurses Association. (2015). *Code of Ethics for Nurses with Interpretive Statements.* Silver Spring, MD: Author.

American Nurses Association. (2016). Incivility, Bullying, and Workplace Violence (website). Retrieved from http://www.nursingworld.org/MainMenuCategories/WorkplaceSafety/Healthy-Nurse/bullyingworkplaceviolence

American Nurses Credentialing Center (ANCC). (2016a). Benefits. Retrieved from http://www.nursecredentialing.org/Magnet/ProgramOverview/WhyBecomeMagnet

American Nurses Credentialing Center (ANCC). (2016b). Homepage. Retrieved from http://www.nursecredentialing.org/Magnet

American Nurses Credentialing Center (ANCC). (2016c). *Magnet Model.* Retrieved from http://www.nursecredentialing.org/Magnet/ProgramOverview/New-Magnet-Model

Blegen, M. A., Goode, C. J., Park, S. H., Vaughn, T., & Spetz, J. (2013). Baccalaureate education in nursing and patient outcomes. *Journal of Nursing Administration, 43*(2), 89–94.

Bonasall, L. (2011). What is shared governance? Last updated August 11, 2011. Retrieved from http://www.nursingcenter.com/ncblog/august-2011/what-is-shared-governance

Cho, E., Sloane, D. M., Kim, E., Kim, S., Choi, M., Yoo, I. Y., ... Aiken, L. H. (2014). Effects of nurse staffing, work environments, and education on patient mortality: An observational study. *International Journal of Nursing Studies, 52*(2).

Fox, K. C. (2010). Mentor program boosts new nurses' satisfaction and lowers turnover rate. *The Journal of Continuing Education in Nursing, 41.7,* 311–316.

Gelinas, L., & Bohlen, C. (2002). The business case for retention. *Journal of Clinical Systems Management, 4*(78), 14–16, 22.

Hess, R., (2004). From bedside to boardroom—Nursing shared governance. *Online Journal of Issues in Nursing, 9*(1), para 4. Retrieved from www.nursingworld.org/MainMenuCategories/ANAMarketplace/ANAPeriodicals/OJIN/TableofContents/Volume92004/No1Jan04/FromBedsidetoBoardroom.aspx

Huey, F. L., & Hartley, S. (1988). What keeps nurses in nursing: 3,500 nurses tell their stories. *American Journal of Nursing, 88,* 181–188.

Kutney-Lee, A., Sloane, D. M., & Aiken, L. H. (2003). An increase in the number of nurses with baccalaureate degrees is linked to lower rates of postsurgery mortality. *Health Affairs, 32*(3), 579–586.

McKinley, M. (2004). Mentoring matters: Creating, connecting, empowering. *AACN Clinical Issues, 15,* 205–214.

Nursing Solutions, Inc. (2016). *2016 national health care retention and RN staffing report.* Retrieved from http://www.nsinursingsolutions.com/Files/assets/library/retention-institute/NationalHealthcareRNRetentionReport2016.pdf

Selected resources about Magnet-designated hospitals outcomes

Aiken, L. H., Sloane, D. M., Lake E. T., & Weber, A. L. (1999). Organization and outcomes of inpatient AIDS care. *Med Care, 37*(8), 760–772.

Aiken, L. H., Smith, H. L., & Lake, E. T. (1994). Lower Medicare mortality rates among a set of hospitals known for good nursing care. *Med Care,* 32(8), 771–787.

Aiken, L. H., Sochalski, J., & Lake, E. T. (2007). Studying outcomes of organizational change in health services. *Med Care, 35,* NS6–N18.

Berquist-Beringer, S., Davidson, J., Agosto, C., Linde, N. K., Abel, M., Spurling, K., ... Christopher, A. (2009). Evaluation of the national database of nursing quality indicators (NDNQI) training program on pressure ulcers. *The Journal of Continuing Education in Nursing, 40*(6), 252–260.

Bates, D. W., Pruess, K., Souney, P., & Platt, R. (1995). Serious falls in hospitalized patients: Correlates and resource utilization. *The American Journal of Medicine, 99*(2), 137–143.

Clarke, S. P., Sloane D. M., & Aiken, L. H. (2002). Effects of hospital staffing and organizational climate on needlestick injuries to nurses. *American Journal of Public Health, 92*(7), 1115–1119.

Dunton, N., Gajewski, B., Klaus, S., & Pierson, B. (2007). The relationship of nursing workforce characteristics to patient outcomes: A study to assess the economic value of nursing staff and registered nurses. *Online Journal of Issues in Nursing, 12*(3). Retrieved from http://www.nursingworld.org/MainMenuCategories/ANAMarketplace/ANAPeriodicals/OJIN/TableofContents/Volume122007/No3Sept07/NursingWorkforceCharacteristics.html

Dunton, N., Gajewski, B., Taunton, R. L., & Moore, J. (2004). Nursing staffing and patient falls in acute care hospital units. *Nursing Outlook, 52*(1), 53–59.

Gardner, J. K., Fogg, L., Thomas-Hawkins, C., & Latham, C. E. (2007). The relationships between nurses' perceptions of the hemodialysis work environment and nurse turnover, patient satisfaction, and hospitalizations. *Nephrology Nursing Journal, 34*(3), 271–281.

Goode, C. & Blegen, M. (2009). The link between nurse staffing and patient outcomes, 2009. National Magnet Conference abstract and presentation at the Magnet Conference in Louisville, KY, October 1–3. Retrieved from http://www.nursinglibrary.org/vhl/handle/10755/182403

Havens, D. S., & Aiken, L. H. (1999). Shaping systems to promote desired outcomes: The Magnet hospital model. *Journal of Nursing Administration, 29*(2), 14–20.

Hitcho, E. B., Krauss, M. J., Birge, S., Clairborne-Dunagan, W., Fischer, I., Johnson, S., ... Fraser, V. J. (2004). Characteristics and circumstances of falls in hospital setting: A prospective analysis. *Journal of General Internal Medicine, 19*(7), 732–739.

Hook, M. L., & Winchel, S. (2006). Fall-related injuries in acute care: Reducing the risk of harm. *MEDSURG Nursing Journal, 15*(6), 370–381.

Jagger, J., Hunt, E. H., & Peatson, R. D. (1990). Estimated cost of needle-stick for six major needled devices. *Infection Control and Hospital Epidemiology, 11*(11), 584–588.

Neisner, J., & Raymond, B. (2002). *Nurse staffing and care delivery models: A review of the evidence.* Retrieved from http://www.kpihp.org/wp-content/uploads/2012/12/nurse_staffing.pdf

Nurmi, I. & Lüthje, P. (2002). Incidence and costs of falls and fall injuries among elderly in institutional care. *Scandinavian Journal of Primary Health Care, 20*(2), 118–122.

Rosenberg, M. C. (2009, Oct. 1–3). *Do Magnet-recognized hospitals provide better care?* Paper presented at the American Nurses Credentialing Center Magnet Conference, Louisville, KY. Abstract retrieved from http://hdl.handle.net/10755/182328

Stone, P. W., & Gershon, R. R. (2006). Nurse work environments and occupational safety in intensive care units. *Policy, Politics, and Nursing Practice, 39*(7–8, Suppl.), S27–34.

Recommended Reading

Admit One: What You Must Know When Going to the Hospital, But No One Actually Tells You by Kati Kleber (http://www.nursesbooks.org/Homepage/Hot-off-the-Press/Admit-One-What-You-Must-Know-When-Going-to-the-Hospital-But-No-One-Actually-Tells-You.aspx)

Becoming Nursey: From Code Blues to Code Browns, How to Care for Your Patients and Yourself by Kati Kleber (http://www.nurseeyeroll.com/buy-my-nursey-book/)

Debriefing as a Supportive Component for Registered Nurses in Transition by J. Shinners, L. Africa and B. Hawkes, published in the *Journal for Nurses in Professional Development, 2*(4), 212–218.

The Florence Prescription: From Accountability to Ownership by Joe Tye (http://theflorencechallenge.com/)

From Novice to Expert: Excellence and Power in Clinical Practice by Patricia Benner (About which: http://currentnursing.com/nursing_theory/Patricia_Benner_From_Novice_to_Expert.html; http://www.nursing-theory.org/theories-and-models/from-novice-to-expert.php)

From Surviving to Thriving: Navigating the First Year of Nursing Practice by Dr. Boychuk Duchscher, PhD, RN and Dr. Marlene Kramer, PhD, RN, FAAN

Inspired Nurse by Rich Bluni (https://www.firestarterpublishing.com/books/individual-books/inspired-nurse)

Nursing by the Numbers is a data- and information-rich career resource from the American Nurses Association. Its many graphs and tables detail RN and APRN employment and compensation, including national salaries, average earnings for hospital staff RNs, predicted employment over the next decade, salary and hiring trends since the end of the recession, and jobs and wages by state (http://www.nursingworld.org/nbn).

Shared Governance, Third Edition: A Practical Approach to Transforming Interprofessional Healthcare by Robert Hess and Diana Swihart (https://hcmarketplace.com/aitdownloadablefiles/download/aitfile/aitfile_id/1609.pdf)

Index